GW01605683

OCCUPATIONAL THERAPY INTERVENTION PROCESS MODEL

A Model for Planning and Implementing Top–down, Client-centered, and Occupation-based Interventions

Anne G. Fisher, ScD, OT, FAOTA
Professor
Division of Occupational Therapy
Department of Community Medicine and Rehabilitation
Umeå University, Sweden

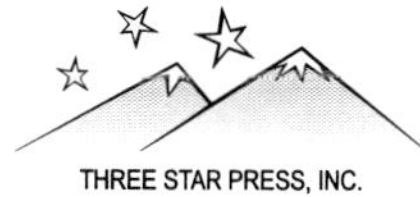

Three Star Press, Inc. • Fort Collins, Colorado • USA

Printed in the United States of America

ISBN 0-9774301-5-4

Published and distributed by Three Star Press, Inc., Fort Collins, Colorado, USA
To purchase additional copies of this publication, contact AMPS Project International at info@ampsintl.com.

CONTRIBUTORS

ANNE G. FISHER, ScD, OT, FAOTA
Professor
Department of Community Medicine and Rehabilitation
Division of Occupational Therapy
Umeå University
Umeå
Sweden

LOU ANN GRISWOLD, PhD, OTR, FAOTA
Associate Professor
College of Health and Human Services
Department of Occupational Therapy
University of New Hampshire
Durham, New Hampshire
USA

ACKNOWLEDGEMENTS

I want to express my appreciation to all those participants in Occupational Therapy Intervention Process Model (OTIPM) courses around the world for your critical comments and questions. They have been an ongoing source of stimulation — your problems and concerns, and the realities of the practice arenas in which you work, have provided an important foundation for many of the changes that have occurred in the OTIPM since it was first published in 1998 (Fisher, 1998).

I also want to thank Michael Munkholm, who has helped me with some of the artwork in this text, in particular, the cover design. His help and his unending patience have been a great source of support.

To those who may ask, "What is the meaning behind the cover design?", perhaps Michael's own words provide the best answer:

For me, when I listen to you and what you do, I get a picture of how OTIPM works. At the center, we have the core — the client — a person or a group of people. The rays represent power or energy. They are the different tools, methods, and routines you use to improve the client's abilities. They go into the client and out again — all that goes in is a potential form of energy for the client. Sometimes, when you work together with the client, what you do does not work, and when that happens, you have to try another strategy.

TABLE OF CONTENTS

LIST OF TABLES

LIST OF FIGURES

LIST OF DOCUMENTATION EXAMPLES

1. INTRODUCTION

The purpose of this text is to present the Occupational Therapy Intervention Process Model (OTIPM) as a way of thinking about occupation and occupational therapy that enables occupational therapists to practice in a manner that stresses our unique focus on occupation. More specifically, "function," from the perspective of occupational therapy, relates primarily to ***the ability of our clients to perform the daily life tasks that they want to perform, need to perform, and/or that they are expected to perform so as to be able to assume desired life roles and level of participation in society***.

The OTIPM, therefore, is based on the assertions that (a) each individual is unique and has the will to engage in activity that yields a sense of meaning and/or purpose for the person engaged in the doing, (b) a client's engagement in occupation (meaningful and purposeful doing) is the central focus our profession, (c) the therapeutic use of occupation is our primary "means" for promoting our clients' abilities to engage in occupation, and (d) our clients achieving engagement in meaningful and purposeful occupation is our primary "end."[1] Through developing the OTIPM, my goal has been to provide occupational therapists with a ***structure to guide our professional reasoning*** as we plan and implement occupational therapy services. More specifically, the OTIPM is a model to guide professional reasoning ***in a manner that ensures that we stress a client-centered, top–down, and occupation-based approach to assessment and intervention***.

In this chapter, I will introduce each of these concepts — *client-centered*, *top–down*, and *occupation-based* approach to assessment and intervention. As part of that discussion, I will present some of the key terminology used in the OTIPM. I will then present a brief overview of the OTIPM, followed by a short discussion of *theory-driven* versus *process-driven reasoning*. I will end this chapter with an overview of the purpose and content of the remaining chapters.

1.1 Client-centered Occupational Therapy

The concept of working with the client in a manner that is client-centered has its origins in the work of Carl Rogers (1951). More recently, the idea of working in a

---

[1] My use of the terms *means* and *end* is based on Trombly Latham (2008b, 2008c; Trombly 1995a) — she used the terms *occupation-as-means*, and *occupation-as-end*.

client-centered manner has also become a central concept within the profession of occupational therapy (Canadian Association of Occupational Therapists [CAOT], 1997, 2002; Fearing & Clark, 2000; Fisher, 1998; Kielhofner, 2002, 2008). Our Canadian colleagues should perhaps be given credit for first articulating the concept of client-centered practice from an occupational therapy perspective (CAOT, 1997, 2002).

To work in a manner that is client-centered involves developing therapeutic rapport and a collaborative relationship with our clients, and then working together with our clients in a manner that stresses the clients' own perspectives. This means that we must make every attempt possible to understand the client and to see the client through the client's own eyes. ***We must also commit to collaborating with our clients to enable them to reach their goals***. An important component is that ***we must always maintain our focus on the client's needs and desires, and ensure that the client is actively involved in making decisions about what services we will provide, how services will be provided, and the formulation of the client's goals and intervention plan*** (American Occupational Therapy Association [AOTA], 2005; Fisher & Nyman, 2007; Förbundet Sveriges Arbetsterapeuter [FSA], 2005).

1.1.1 Meet the Client "Where the Client Is"

To work in a manner that is client-centered involves meeting the client "where the client is" in terms of the client's (a) self-reported needs and desires, (b) level of motivation, and/or (c) understanding and insight into whatever problems with occupational performance the client currently has or may have in the future. Importantly, it also means ***honoring and respecting the client's perspective and goals, and not taking away the client's dreams***.

I once worked with a young man who had had a high level spinal cord injury. He used a wheelchair as he was unable to walk, and while he had active control of elbow flexion and wrist extension, but he had no active control of his finger movements. When I first met him, he told me that his goal was to return to his family's business and work as a roofer. His prognosis for recovery of active control of his arms and legs was poor; he had been told by his doctor about his condition and that he would never be able to walk again. Perhaps he had not heard what his doctor had said, or perhaps he was in "denial of his problems." It did not matter. I knew that it was important to not take away his dreams as they were an important source of his motivation. Instead of saying to him, "You will not be able to do that, you cannot walk," I chose to respect his dreams, and use them as a means of collaborating with him to develop relevant short term goals that were more realistic, but which might move him closer to a potential longer term goal of gainful employment. Even if he never was able to walk again, I knew that he might, if interested in doing so, be able to return to his family business in some other role than as a roofer (e.g., in a management role). What was critical in the process of our developing rapport and a sound collaborative relationship was to take his lead, and not impose on him my own views of what I thought might be realistic. After all, I had no crystal ball to be able to know what his future might bring.

1.1.2 Who Is the Client?

To fully understand the idea of working in a manner that is client-centered, it is important to consider: Who is the client? I use term ***client*** broadly to refer to the person, family, organization, or other constellation or group of persons for whom intervention is considered. More specifically, I use three different terms to refer to the "client" (Fisher & Nyman, 2007):

1. ***Person*** — most commonly, the person who seeks or was referred for occupational therapy services (e.g., patient, customer, consumer, student), including well persons who seek preventative occupational therapy services.

2. ***Client constellation*** — both the person who seeks/was referred for occupational therapy services and others who live with, work with, or are otherwise closely connected to the person who seeks/was referred for occupational therapy services, provided they also experience problems with occupational performance is relation to living or working with the person who seeks/was referred for occupational therapy services. Examples include (a) a man who has had a stroke and his close family members who live with him, (b) a woman with dementia who is attending a day treatment center and the staff who are working with her on a regular basis, or (c) a student in an elementary classroom and his or her teacher. Again, it is critical to stress is that ***only those other persons who are experiencing problems of occupational performance in relation to working or interacting with the person who seeks/was referred for occupational therapy services are included in the client constellation.***

3. ***Client group*** — a group of persons who share similar occupational performance problems, but who otherwise are not related, nor have a close relationship with each other. Examples of client groups include (a) the ward personnel who are responsible for caring for persons living in a nursing home, whether it be a specific

person, or all who live there; (b) a group of persons with developmental disabilities who participate in a group intervention program at a day treatment center; (c) a group of students who all receive occupational therapy services together within a classroom setting; (d) a company (i.e., a client group that might include administrators as well as a group of employees); and (e) a population of persons living within a geographic region (e.g., well older adults living in a large city).

I will use the term ***client*** when the person or persons to which I am referring may be any one of the three "types" of clients — the person who seeks/was referred for occupational therapy services, the client constellation, or a client group. For example, earlier, I referred to "the ability of our clients to perform the daily life tasks that they want and need to perform." By doing so, my deliberate intent was to specify that the persons to which I am referring may be the person who seeks/was referred for occupational therapy services, others in the client constellation, and/or a group of persons who comprise a client group.

Ultimately, ***the determination of who is the client is based on knowing who has expressed concern about or is experiencing problems with performing their daily life tasks, those performed in connection with the person who seeks/was referred for occupational therapy services***. For example, if a person with a disability lacks motivation for occupational performance, or for some other reason has limited ability to recognize the meaning and purpose of occupation (including the social relevance of the daily life tasks in question), it is likely that someone else in that person's client constellation is having to care for that person, and that the caregiver is also experiencing needs related to those occupational performances connected with his or her caregiver role. It becomes our role, therefore, to determine whether or not the caregiver has any concerns about, and/or is experiencing any problems with, carrying out his or her role as caregiver. If there are no concerns or problems, occupational therapy services may not be indicated, and that person is ***not*** a member of the client constellation. If there are concerns or problems, then our intervention must include, and may best be directed toward, the caregiver and those caregiving tasks that have meaning and purpose to the caregiver.

In this process, however, ***we must not forget to consider that the person who seeks/was referred for occupational therapy services is always a primary component of whom we define as our client***. Even if he or she is not able to express them, we must also consider his or her meanings and purposes as best we can via information we can gather from those who know the person and are familiar with his or her prior (and potential future) circumstances, desires, and needs.

1.1.3 Some "Words of Warning" Related to Working in a Manner that is Client-centered

Working in a manner that is truly client-centered is not always easy. On one hand, we are challenged to place the client's needs and desires in the center and to understand them from the client's perspective. This means that when we work with clients who for some reason are not able to express their concerns, perspectives, and/or goals, we must constantly remain alert to the risk that we, other professionals, or others in the person's client constellation may be tempted to make decisions for the person that are not based on what the person would want if he or she could express them. At the same time, we have a responsibility to not support clients who express needs or desires that would be unethical to support. That is, to ***practice in a manner that is client-centered does not mean that we do whatever the client wants***. The setting where we work may limit what services we can provide (e.g., if we are employed in a public school in the US, we are mandated by law to only provide services that support the student in his or her student role) (Individuals with Disabilities Education Improvement Act of 2004 [IDEA]).

Another caution pertains to our ***ethical responsibility to retain the focus of our practice on occupation***. I often meet occupational therapists who tell me that their client's goals are often related to improvement of hand strength, capacity to walk, or other underlying body functions. They then ask me, "If I am to work in a client-centered manner, and improvement of body functions is the client's goal, why is it not appropriate for me to use hand strengthening exercises or other similar interventions as my 'occupational' therapy?" In such cases, if we are to truly practice in a manner that is client-centered, we must clarify our role, and redirect the client to those occupational performances that might be impacted by the client's underlying impairments. If we are successful in redirecting the client, and enabling the client to identify those task performances that are impacted by the underlying impairments, we can then implement restorative occupation to address concerns that have been targeted by the client. ***If the client persists with a focus on underlying impairments and declines those services we can ethically offer, we have a professional obligation to decline to offer services (at least until the client identifies occupation-related needs), and to refer the client to other professionals who are most qualified to treat the underlying impairments using the forms of therapy the client is willing to accept*** (e.g., physical therapy).

1.2 Top–down Occupational Therapy Evaluation

When the OTIPM is used to guide our professional reasoning process as we evaluate our clients, we use ***a true top–down approach***. The reason for this is to avoid (a) using a top–to–bottom–up approach and jumping too quickly to interpreting the cause of the client's problems; and/or (b) using a bottom–up approach, and focusing first on the client's impairments and body function limitations that are assumed to limit occupational performance. I will describe each of these approaches below.

1.2.1 Top–down Approach

When using an top–down approach, the occupational therapist begins with a broad picture of who is the client, what are the client's needs and desires, and which tasks does the client want to be able to perform so as to be able to assume desired life roles in a manner that brings satisfaction, and which support the client's desired level of participation in society. In this process, it is also important to determine what task performances the client identifies as limiting the ability to assume life roles and participation in society (see Figure 1).

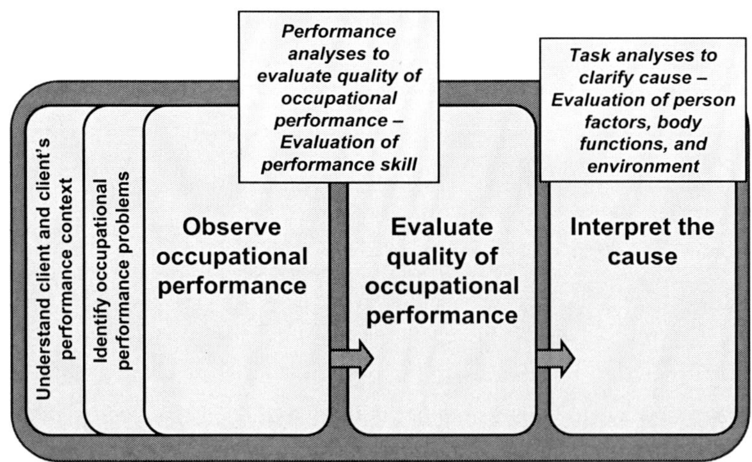

Figure 1. **Top–down reasoning: Initial phases of the evaluation process.**

Once a broad picture, from the perspective of the client, is obtained, the occupational therapist focuses next on observing the client perform tasks that the client has identified as a problem. The goal of the observation of the client's task performance is to identify which performance skills (i.e., actions, smallest observable units of occupation) were effective and which were not. Only when the occupational therapist has determined which performance skills were effective or ineffective does the occupational therapist proceed to consider the reasons for, or causes of, the client's diminished quality of occupational performance (e.g., person factors, body functions, environmental factors) (see Figure 1). When working in a true top–down manner, the occupational therapist then collaborates with the client to formulate goals based on the results of the evaluation of the client's quality of performance of desired tasks. Finally, based on the findings of this top–down evaluation process, the client and the occupational therapist work together to plan and implement occupation-based interventions.

1.2.2 Bottom–up Approach

In contrast to a top–down approach, when an occupational therapist uses a bottom–up approach, he or she ***begins with a focus on the evaluation of the client's person factors, body functions, and/or environmental factors***. Those that are found to be "diminished" in some way are then viewed as the cause of the client's problems with performance of daily life tasks (see Figure 2). One problem with working in this manner is that the occupational therapist risks planning and implementing interventions focused on person factors, impairments of body functions, and/or environmental constraints without consideration of who is this client, and what needs and desires the client has for enhanced occupation.

Another problem is that the occupational therapist does not evaluate the quality of the client's task performances, and instead focuses on person factors (e.g., habits, routines, values) and/or impairments of underlying neuromuscular, biomechanical, cognitive, or psychosocial body functions. Yet, the best available evidence has shown that interventions focused on person factors and remediation of impairments of body functions are not only time-consuming, they also have a limited impact with regard to improvements of occupational performance. That is, research has failed to demonstrate a strong enough relationship between body functions and occupational performance to support the basic assumption that if the underlying cause of limitations in occupational performance can be identified and treated, then the effects will generalize to improved occupational performance (Bernspång, Asplund, Eriksson, & Fugl-Meyer, 1987;

Jongbloed, Brighton, & Stacey, 1988; Judge, Schechtman, Cress, & the FICSIT Group, 1996; Lichtenberg & Nanna, 1994; Pincus et al., 1989; Reed, Jagust, & Seab, 1989; Skurla, Rogers, & Sunderland, 1988; Teri, Borson, Kiyak, & Yamagishi, 1989; Trombly Latham, 2008c). Additional evidence lies in studies which indicate that the effectiveness of restorative approaches may be limited (Benedict et al., 1994; Fetters & Kluzik, 1996; Hutzler, Chacham, Bergman, & Szeinberg, 1998; Kaplan, Polatajko, Wilson, & Faris, 1993; Law et al., 1997; Nakayama, Jørgensen, Raaschou, & Olsen, 1994; Neistadt, 1992). There exist many additional studies that are not cited here, including meta-analyses, that occupational therapists are encouraged to search for and critically review based on their own evidence-based practice research questions. The ones I have included are merely intended to show the broad range of areas of practice where existing evidence does not support our common assumptions.

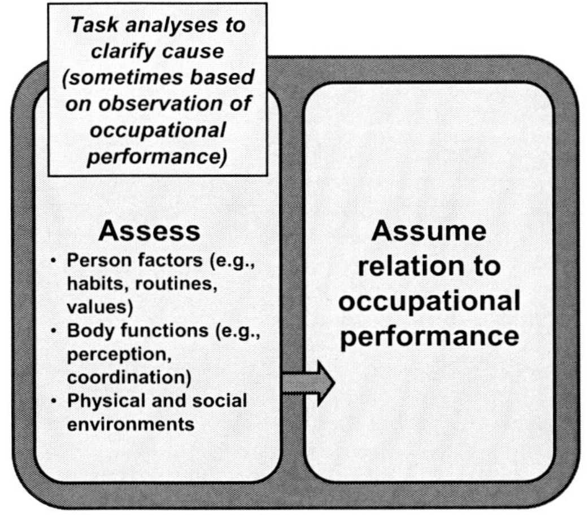

Figure 2. **Bottom–up reasoning evaluation process.**

1.2.3 Top–to–bottom–up Approach

Still another approach often used in occupational therapy I refer to as a top–to–bottom–up approach. In the literature, this approach is often referred to as a top–down approach because the occupational therapist begins the evaluation process by determining who is the client and/or what are the client's occupation-related needs and desires (cf. CAOT, 2002; Fearing & Clark, 2000; Kielhofner, 2008). With this approach, however, there is often an over-reliance and "trust" in the client's ability to self-report what he or she can or cannot do effectively. The occupational therapist also does not take the needed time to (a) adequately verify the client's self-reported problems through observation, and (b) identify the specific performance skills that actually are ineffective. Instead, and the reason for the name I have given to this approach, the ***occupational therapist proceeds directly from the client's self-report (i.e., top) to the determination of what person factors, body functions, and/or environmental factors (i.e., bottom) may be the cause of the client's problems performing daily life tasks (i.e., back to the top)*** (see Figure 3).

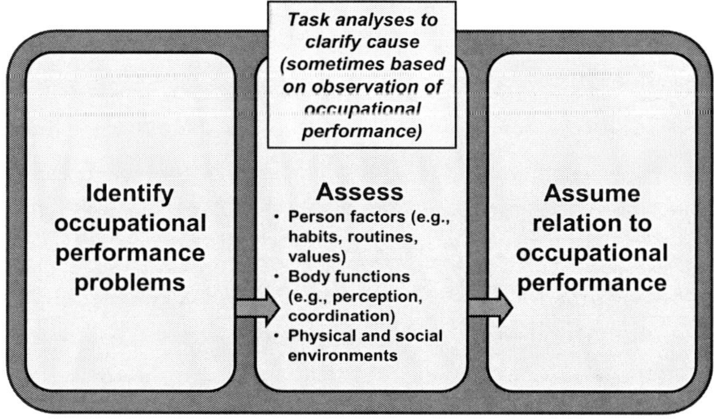

Figure 3. **Top–to–bottom–up reasoning evaluation process.**

While Trombly Latham (2008a) also claims to use a top–down approach to assessment, and her model is perhaps the one that most closely approximates a true top–down reasoning process, careful analysis reveals that even her approach remains top–to–bottom–up. That is, she states that performance of life roles is dependent upon underlying capacities, and she considers performance skills to be equivalent to underlying body functions such as strength and memory. Thus, there appears to be no performance analysis (as defined within the OTIPM) before progressing to determination of the cause.

1.3 Occupation-based Evaluation and Intervention

I noted earlier that our client's engagement in occupation (meaningful and purposeful activity) is the central focus our profession, and that the therapeutic use of occupation is our primary "means" for promoting our clients' abilities to engage in occupation. ***If the focus of our practice is to be occupation, we must assure that the focus of our evaluations, interventions, and documentation, not just the outcome ("end"), also are occupation.*** Moreover, not only should our evaluations and interventions be focused on occupation, they must emphasize the use of occupation-based methods. That is, while many occupational therapists sometimes justify what they do with the claim that their methods are designed to promote our "end" — our clients achieving engagement in occupation — my premise is that if we are to practice as ***occupational*** therapists (and not ***physical*** therapists, ***psycho***therapists, etc.), we must also evaluate our client's in the context of occupational performance, and then use occupation as our primary form of therapy — we must implement ***occupational*** therapy. Moreover, if we want to know if our clients have problems engaging in meaningful and purposeful activity and performing the daily life tasks they need and want to perform, we must evaluate both their quality of occupational performance as well and their degree of satisfaction with their occupational performances (e.g., satisfaction with quality of occupational performance, satisfaction with level of engagement or participation). ***Both the "insider," client perspective, based on self-report; and the "outsider" perspective, based on observation of engagement in occupation, are critical.***

1.3.1 Definitions of Some Key Terms

As part of understanding the idea of occupation-based evaluation and intervention, it is important to examine more closely the meanings of some the terms I have been using: (a) ***occupation***, ***task***, and ***activity***; and (b) ***meaning*** and ***purpose***. The reason for this is that in both our common, "everyday" languages and in occupational therapy literature, we often use terms in a manner that leads to confusion. For example, it is common to think that the terms *activity* and *task* are synonyms. Yet, while their definitions overlap to a small degree, to a much greater extent, they actually differ from one another.[2] In occupational therapy literature, it is also common to equate the terms

[2] When I teach courses in countries were English is not the primary language, occupational therapists often argue, "But, in our language, they really are synonyms." Yet, when I look them up in dictionaries, I find that the same problem invariably exists in other languages, just as it does in English. For my Scandinavian colleagues, I use the example of the Swedish terms *uppgift* [task] and *aktivitet* [activity].

task and *occupation* and/or to use them interchangeably (cf. CAOT, 2002), even though they differ in fundamental ways (Fisher, 2006b). Finally, in some languages, the term *activity* must be used as a synonym for *occupation* (e.g., Scandinavian languages) (cf. Fisher & Nyman, 2007). When this occurs without the simultaneous use of adjectives such as "meaningful" or "purposeful," the difference between *activity* (simply doing something, but without engagement) and *occupation* (being engaged in doing something that has meaning and/or purpose for the doer) becomes obscured.

1.3.2 Occupation

In the *Oxford English Dictionary* (1989), *occupation* is defined as ***the action of seizing, taking possession of, or occupying space or time.***[3] It is also defined as ***the holding of positions*** — as in one's roles. Finally, occupation is defined as a ***series of actions in which one is engaged.*** Therefore, when the term *occupation* is used properly, it clearly pertains to the carrying out of actions, doing something, and being engaged that doing. The "something" that the person is engaged in may be writing a letter, driving a bus, playing football, listening to a radio, or putting on one's shirt. In the OTIPM, therefore, I use the term *occupation* (and occupational performance) to refer to a person's ***engagement in a process*** — the process of writing the letter, driving the bus, playing football, listening to the radio, or putting on one's shirt. Finally, engagement occurs because what the person does has associated with it some form of meaning and/or purpose.

I refer to it as an engagement in a process because the person must perform a series of goal-directed actions over time in order to enact occupational performances. In the

---

Closer examination of the core meanings of these two terms reveals that they are actually more different than they are similar, despite our imprecise use of them as synonyms in our "everyday" Swedish language.

[3] While the term *occupation* was originally used in the United States to name our profession, other terms have been used in other countries to replace the term *occupation*. For example, in Europe, terms that refer to work (e.g., *ergo*, *arbete*) have been used in place of occupation. The use of these terms may be due to the fact that in English, occupation is commonly used to refer to one's work, job, and/or profession, a use that does not convey the true essence of our profession. Yet, it may be that it was this meaning of the term that provided the basis for translating occupation from English into a term that refers to work. It also may be that there was a deliberate desire to avoid the use of the term *occupation* because, in some languages, the term is used almost exclusively to refer to the occupation of space in a military sense (e.g., to invade, to occupy, to seize land occupied by others), and hence, it may connote a more negative meaning than desired. Yet, it is this very meaning of the term *occupation* that we should think of when we use it to refer to our profession and to what people do. People seize, take possession of, or occupy time, space, and roles, in an active but more neutral (nonmilitary) sense (e.g., "to occupy a room"). Whatever term has been adopted in other countries, it is important to be aware of the root meaning and the "power" of the original name given our profession — *occupational* therapy.

OTIPM, I call these actions ***performance skills***.[4] They are referred to as skills because they are ***the smallest observable units of occupation***, and each action we observe a person perform may be more or less skilled.

If we examine more closely the idea that occupation refers to the action of seizing, taking possession of, or occupying ***space***, we can think of the actions (and task performances) our clients must perform to occupy their homes, their schools, their workplaces, and the places where they engage in recreation or leisure activities. Similarly, when we speak of the action of seizing, taking possession of, or occupying ***time***, we can think about our client's need to occupy time, not just in the sense of "being busy," but also in a sense that connotes the action of carrying out daily life task performances that are meaningful and purposeful from the perspective of the person. That is, when we occupy time, we engage in something. Even when we might want to think of it as "doing nothing" (e.g., listening to the radio, sitting under a tree and watching the clouds pass overhead), we engage in a course of actions (a process) that unfold over time (e.g., walking over and turning on the radio, selecting the station, adjusting the volume, and then walking back, sitting down in a comfortable chair, and listening to the radio). And lastly, when we speak of the action of seizing, taking possession of, or occupying (i.e., holding) ***roles***, we can think about the task performances our clients must enact in order to assume their life roles in a manner that the clients perceive as having meaning and purpose, and which support their desired level of participation in society.

1.3.3 Activity versus Task

In the dictionary, the definition of the term ***activity*** pertains to action (i.e., the state of being active, active doing) (Merriam-Webster, 1996), and in occupational therapy, that action is most commonly observed in the context of daily life task performances. In contrast, the term ***task*** is properly used to refer to a specified or defined piece of work that is to be done (Merriam-Webster, 1996). Despite the fact that we often use the terms *task* and *activity* as if they were synonymous, the task is *what* is done; whereas, activity refers to the *actions* we can observe people performing as they carry out that task performances. Said in slightly different words, ***the term* activity *pertains to the actions we observe (i.e., doing, task performances); whereas, the term* task *refers to***

---

[4] The first use of term *performance skills* to describe observable actions of performance emerged during the development of the Assessment of Motor and Process Skills (Fisher, 1989), and began with a collaborative dialogue between Gary Kielhofner and myself. That process is described in more detail in Chapter 6.

what the person will do, or what he or she has done after the activity ceases. When activity is meaningful and purposeful, we call it occupation (Fisher, 1998).

Keeping in mind that ***what will be (or what was) done is the task***, and ***what we observe is action or activity***, we can think about an example. A person might say to us, "This morning I got dressed and ate breakfast. This evening, I plan to socialize with friends and watch football on television." This person is speaking, talking about something, but we are not able to see him getting dressed, eating breakfast, socializing with his friends, or watching football on television because it happened before we met him or will happen later in the day. Clearly, we do not see the action or activity. Thus, the proper term to use is *task*. If, on the other hand, I am observing this man as he is getting dressed, then I am observing action or activity — I see him ***doing*** it — I can observe the ***chain of actions he performs*** as he goes through the process of getting dressed.

1.3.4 Meaning and Purpose

Recall that the definition of occupation stressed the idea of being engaged in action. Engagement comes from a sense of meaning and/or purpose derived from or experienced during the doing. ***Meaning*** pertains to the significance of the task to the person and the experiences the person associates with the task performances. The meaning provides a source of motivation for occupational performance. ***Purpose*** pertains to the person's aim, intended goal, or reason for doing; a sense of purpose helps to organize occupational performance (Trombly, 1995a). Moreover, the meaning is often derived from the purpose and vice versa (Fisher, 1998) (see Figure 4). This perspective, that meaning and purpose are interrelated, and that neither is viewed as "the one" that always precedes the other, is a unique feature of the OTIPM.

When we consider meaning and purpose in this manner, we are free to acknowledge that ***the meaningfulness of the doing can be derived from extrinsic sources (aims, goals, end-products) and/or from intrinsic sources (experiences)***. If the occupational performance is preparing a gourmet meal, an example of an ***extrinsic*** source of motivation is the person's aim to get the meal prepared and then share it with a friend. Examples of ***intrinsic*** sources of motivation include the enjoyment of preparing the gourmet meal and the experience of pleasure when eating the meal with a friend. When we say that purpose can be derived from the meaning and vice versa, we can see that wanting to prepare a meal for a friend and experiencing the pleasure of eating with a friend can be both the purpose and the meaning. Which came first would be determined based on the primary source of motivation. That is, did purpose precede meaning or did meaning precede purpose? Said in other words, did the person first have the idea that it would be nice to have a chance to eat dinner together with a friend, and hence, become engaged in the enjoyment of preparing the meal; or did he first have a desire to prepare the meal for the shear enjoyment of cooking, so he decided to invite over the friend to eat the meal?

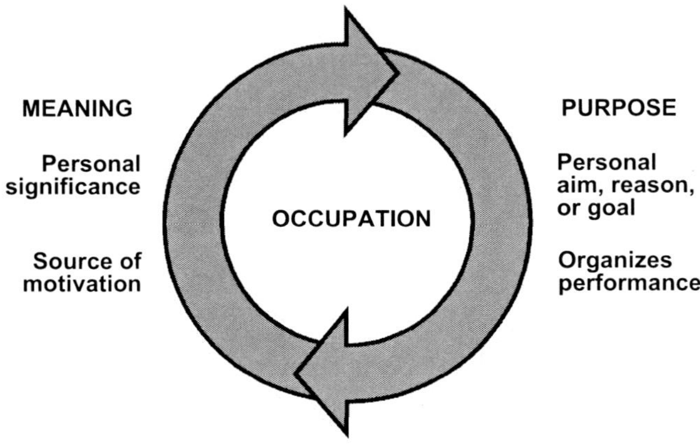

Figure 4. **Interrelationship between the meaning and the purpose of occupation.**

As we consider the issue of meaning and purpose, we must also consider those persons who lack motivation for occupational performance or who have diminished awareness of their disabilities. These persons may fail to find meaning and purpose in those tasks performances they used to perform or that they are expected to perform by society. How do we engage such persons in occupation — task performances that a person perceives as having meaning and purpose — if the person perceives no meaning or purpose? There is no easy answer to that question; determining what activities are of interest to the client and that the client perceives as having meaning and/or purpose can be one of our greatest challenges. Yet, finding that "spark of motivation" can make the critical difference (see Fortmeier & Thanning , 1998 for an example).

1.4 Overview of the OTIPM

When we use the OTIPM to guide true top–down evaluation and then plan and implement occupation-based interventions, we must begin by simultaneously establishing the ***client-centered performance context***[5] and beginning the ongoing process of developing ***therapeutic rapport*** (see Figure 5). Establishing therapeutic rapport provides the foundation for our ongoing ***collaborative relationships*** with our clients. This means that we focus first on understanding the client, the context of the client's occupational performance, and the ability of our clients to perform the daily life tasks that they want, need, and/or are expected to perform to be able to fulfill their roles competently and with satisfaction. That is, one goal of establishing the client-centered performance context is to find out as much as we can about the client (e.g., relevant roles and related task performances, level of motivation, interests, routines, age), the physical and social environments where the client's occupational performances take place, relevant societal factors, and so on. After we have gathered this information (i.e., ***resources and limitations with the client-centered performance context***), we can summarize and document what contextual factors support or facilitate the client's occupational performance and which may be hindering or limiting the client's occupational performance. When we consider occupational therapy services focused on prevention and wellness, we also consider what factors may emerge and begin to limit occupational performance.

Another goal of establishing the client-centered performance context is to determine what tasks are meaningful and purposeful to the client and which of those the client self-reports that the person and/or others in the client constellation do or do not perform competently and with satisfaction. Again, when the focus of our services is directed toward prevention and wellness, we also consider tasks the client risks performing less competently and/or with diminished satisfaction.

Among those tasks that the client reports as not performing competently or with satisfaction, the occupational therapist also determines which task performances the client wants to prioritize for further evaluation and as possible foci of intervention (i.e., ***identify and prioritize reported strengths and problems of occupational performance***). Based on this information, the occupational therapist documents which occupational performances are ***self-reported strengths*** and which are ***self-reported problems***, as

[5] As will be discussed further in Chapter 4, the context includes not only external factors associated with the task and the physical and social environments; it also includes factors internal to the person, including personal factors and body functions.

expressed by the person and/or others in the client constellation. Those problems that the client prioritizes for further evaluation not only become potential foci for intervention, they will also likely be targeted in the client's goals as they are developed collaboratively with the occupational therapist.

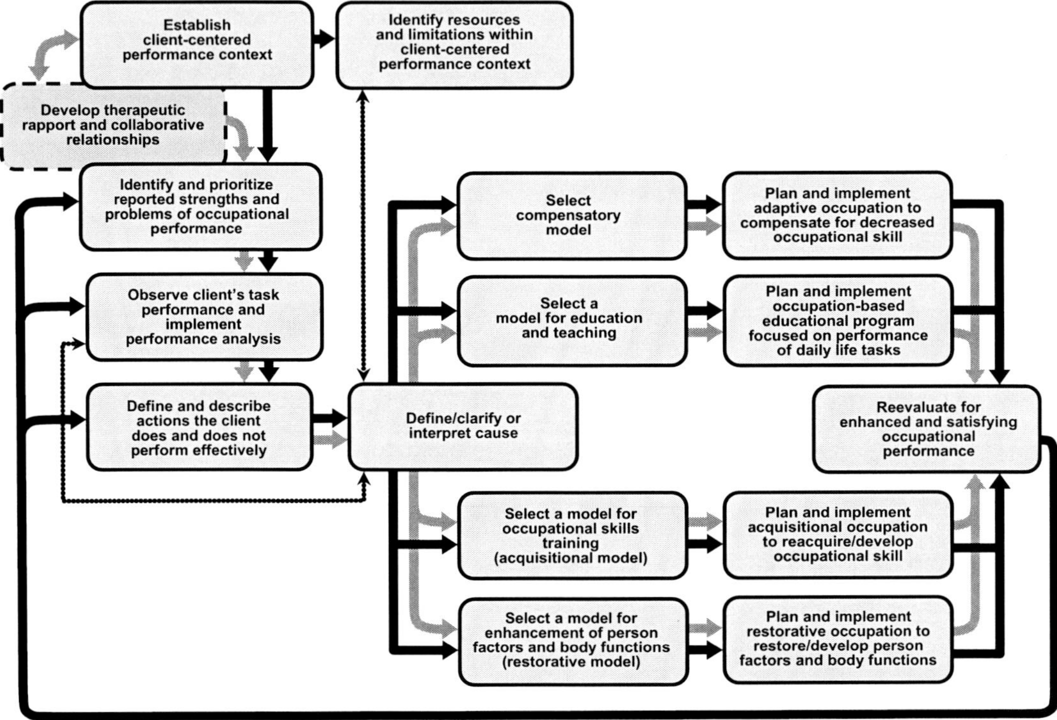

Figure 5. **Occupational Therapy Intervention Process Model.**

Then, having begun the ongoing process of developing therapeutic rapport and collaborative relationships (schematically represented by the grey arrows that extend throughout the intervention process in Figure 5), and knowing what task performances have been prioritized for further evaluation by the client and are potential foci for intervention, the occupational therapist ***observes the client's task performances and implements performance analyses***. Implementing performance analyses are a critical and unique feature of the OTIPM. A performance analysis is the observational evaluation of the quality of a person's occupational performance. The outcome of a performance analysis is for the occupational therapist to (a) ***define and describe those goal-directed actions of occupational performanc***e (i.e., motor, process, and/or social interaction performance skills) ***the person did and did not perform effectively***, and (b) document the person's occupational performance in terms of the quality of those goal-directed actions that comprised the occupational performance. It is important to stress that the implementation of a performance analysis requires that the occupational therapist observe the quality of the goal-directed actions within the context of the person and/or others in the client constellation performing naturalistic daily life tasks that are relevant to and prioritized by those who perform the tasks. Even when occupational therapy services are directed toward prevention and wellness, the observation of prioritized tasks is critical. Moreover, when prevention or wellness programs are to be implemented for the benefit of populations, representative persons in the target group can be interviewed and observed. Depending on the target group, those representatives should include persons who are beginning to demonstrate or experience the problems for which the preventative or wellness programs are to be implemented.

In the true top–down evaluation process defined in the OTIPM, it is not until ***after*** the occupational therapist has defined and described the quality (i.e., level of effort, efficiency, safety, independence, and/or social appropriateness) of the goal-directed actions of a particular task performance that the occupational therapist proceeds to ***define/clarify or interpret the cause*** of the person's problems of occupational performance. The "cause" (or anticipated cause) may be related to (a) the personal characteristics of the person (e.g., impairments and body function limitations, person factors), (b) physical or social environments, and/or (c) societal factors. As with each preceding step, our interpretation of the cause may be included in our documentation, but only ***after*** we have documented occupational performance. That is, we want to stress "occupation-first" documentation.

Again, these steps of implementing a performance analysis and describing the quality of the goal-directed actions of task performance ***before*** defining/clarifying or interpreting the cause of the person's problems of occupational performance are critical steps that ensure true top–down and occupation-based evaluation and intervention. They are steps that are not considered in other so-called top–down approaches described in the literature (cf. CAOT, 2002, Fearing & Clark, 2000). When they are mentioned, they are to be implemented simultaneously with evaluation of the cause (e.g., person factors, body functions; environment) (AOTA, 2002; Kielhofner, 2008; Trombly Latham, 2008a).

It is only ***after*** the occupational therapist (a) implements one or more performance analyses, (b) describes the goal-directed actions of performance that the client did and did not perform effectively, and (c) defines/clarifies the cause of the client's problems with occupational performance, that the initial evaluation phase of the intervention process is complete. Sometime during the evaluation phase of the OTIPM, the client's goals must also be established and documented. Once the client's goals are established, and the evaluation phase in completed, the occupational therapist ***selects which model or models of practice to use to plan and implement occupation-based intervention***. This is in contrast to most process-oriented models which specify that the occupational therapist is to select a model for intervention ***before*** initiating the evaluation process (cf. CAOT, 2002; Pedretti & Zoltan, 1990; Reed & Sanderson, 1999).

The model(s) selected for planning and implementing intervention can be focused on compensation, acquisition, restoration, and/or education and teaching (see Figure 5). Occupation-based activities used with each model are discussed in more detail in Chapter 2, and the therapeutic principles of each of these models are discussed in more detail in Chapter 3. Briefly, these models and their associated intervention strategies are as follows:

1. ***Adaptive occupation*** — therapeutic use of occupation that involves adapted methods of doing, adaptive equipment and assistive technology, and modifications to the physical and social environments to enhance quality of performance of daily life tasks and engagement in daily life. Adaptive occupation always includes collaborative consultation and the use of educational strategies associated with (a) provision of recommendations and/or determination of what adaptations to introduce, and (b) training in their safe and effective use.

2. ***Acquisitional occupation*** — therapeutic use of occupation designed to enable clients to reacquire or develop occupational skill (i.e., occupational skills or activity training) in order to (a) restore occupational skill among clients who have lost their abilities to perform daily life tasks; (b) develop occupational skill among clients who have never acquired their abilities to perform daily life tasks, or (c) maintain, prevent loss of, or enhance occupational skill among clients who may be at risk for loss of their abilities to perform daily life tasks. Acquisitional occupation is ***focused directly on restoring, developing, maintaining, preventing loss of, or enhancing the client's quality of occupational performance***, and always includes collaborative consultation and the use of educational strategies

associated with (a) the provision of recommendations and/or determination of what forms of occupational skills or activity training to introduce, and (b) the provision of such training.

3. ***Restorative occupation*** — therapeutic use of occupation designed to facilitate (a) restoration of person factors (e.g., habits, routines, values) and lost body functions (including motivation); (b) development of person factors and/or body functions that have never been acquired; or (c) maintenance, prevention of loss, or enhancement of person factors and/or body functions among clients who may be at risk for loss of underlying capacities. Restorative occupation is ***focused toward restoring, developing, maintaining, preventing loss of, or enhancing those person factors or underling body functions thought to underlie occupation***, and always includes consultation and the use of educational strategies associated with (a) provision of recommendations and/or determination of what person factors or body functions training to introduce, and (b) the provision of such training.

4. ***Occupation-based education programs*** — planning and implementation of education programs (i.e., seminars, lectures, workshops) for large groups that are focused on discussion of their daily lives and related occupational performances. An example of such a program would be to organize a program for the families/caregivers of persons with dementia that focuses on (a) the problems of everyday doing experienced by persons with dementia, and (b) how the families/caregivers might build more structure and supports into the caregiving process. Unlike adaptive, acquisitional, and restorative occupation, clients may be given opportunities to discuss possible strategies, but because of the more classroom-like format, no opportunity to practice and learn them is provided during the education program. This does not mean that clients are not encouraged to later try new strategies that they have learned during the education program.

After implementing such interventions, the final step is to implement a follow-up evaluation and ***reevaluate for enhanced and satisfying occupational performance***. Establishing and documenting the client's baseline level of performance (the observed quality of occupational performance), the client's goals, and the outcomes of intervention become the ***basis for evaluating the effectiveness of an occupational therapy program and evidence-based practice***.

1.5 Theory-driven versus Process-driven Reasoning

Hagedorn (1995) differentiates between *theory-driven* and *process-driven* patterns for planning and implementing occupational therapy intervention. When a ***theory-driven*** pattern of reasoning is used, a model or frame of reference is selected at the beginning of the process and is then used "as a conceptual lens which alters and colours all subsequent clinical reasoning and therapeutic actions" (p. 40). The advantage of such an approach is that the professional reasoning of the occupational therapist is simplified and the intervention process may be accelerated. The disadvantage is that the occupational therapist necessarily adopts a more narrow perspective, and, as a result, may ignore information or methods that are beneficial, but that do not fit the model of practice selected.

When a ***process-driven*** pattern of reasoning is used, the decision as to what model(s) to use "is postponed until sufficient information has been gathered and evaluated . . . to enable a decision to be made about the nature of the problem, the intervention required and the selection of a suitable treatment method and medium" (Hagedorn, 1995, p. 40). A process-driven approach is closer to the pattern of reasoning we use when we use the OTIPM. That is, as will be discussed in more detail in Chapter 4, the occupational therapist will link to other conceptual models of practice during the process of establishing the client-centered performance context, when defining/clarifying or interpreting the cause of the person's problems of occupational performance, and/or when planning and implementing intervention. In such instances, however, the occupational therapist does not do so with the specific intention of always using the same model(s) to, for example, interpret the cause and as a guide to planning and implementing intervention.

1.6 Summary and Purpose

Adaptive occupation, acquisitional occupation, and restorative occupation, when based on performance analyses and a true top–down and occupation-based approach to assessment and intervention, are the ***very essence of occupational therapy***. When occupational therapists use evaluation, intervention, and documentation strategies that reflect our unique focus on occupation, we more readily convey to our clients and health care payers[6] that ***we possess unique expertise within the health care arena.***

If occupational therapists are to be fully recognized as uniquely qualified to respond to increasing demands for cost-effective intervention and prevention programs designed to improve and maintain the functional status and the quality of life of our clients, we must be prepared to use assessment, intervention, and documentation methods that reflect the unique perspective of occupational therapy. Our assessment, intervention, and documentation methods, therefore, must emphasize the ability to do and must place doing within a client-centered and *true* top–down context that begins with a thorough understanding of the client, the client's performance context, and those socially- and culturally-relevant occupations that are perceived as meaningful and purposeful by the client. Finally, instead of focusing on the "something we do" (outcome), we must focus on the "doing of something" (process). ***We must observe clients doing to be able to evaluate occupation, and we must intervene both to enhance the effectiveness of the client's doing and the client's satisfaction with that doing — the client's occupational performance.***

The OTIPM provides the occupational therapist with a conceptual structure for linking related knowledge and models of practice to the core knowledge of our profession. The OTIPM also serves as a guide to professional reasoning as we plan and implement occupational therapy assessments and interventions. To this end, I present in Chapter 2 an overview of the types of activities occupational therapists may be observed using as interventions with their clients. Included in Chapter 2 are more comprehensive definitions of adaptive occupation, acquisitional occupation, and restorative occupation. These are the legitimate activities for occupational therapy intervention[7] In Chapter 3, I present the related principles of intervention and the assumptions we make about people when we use the OTIPM. Specific principles are included for applications of the compensatory model, acquisitional and restorative models or approaches, and occupation-based education programs, including related principles for education and consultation. In Chapters 4 and 5, I present the OTIPM in more detail, using two case examples to demonstrate its application in practice. Finally, in Chapter 6, I present a taxonomy of motor, process, and social interaction skills that

---

[6] I have used the term *health care payers* in a generic sense to refer to insurance companies, managed care providers, government agencies, or other organizations that pay for health care or occupational therapy services.

[7] As discussed further in Chapter 2, my use of the term *legitimate activities* should not be confused with what Mosey (1986) referred to as the *legitimate tools* of occupational therapy.

comprise the goal-directed actions of occupational performances that can be evaluated during performance analyses. Each performance skill is defined, and qualitative scales for judging the client's observed level of skill are summarized.

2. TYPES OF INTERVENTIONS USED BY OCCUPATIONAL THERAPISTS

Since the beginning of our profession, occupation has been viewed as both a means and an end (Clark, 1917; Dunton, 1928; Gritzer & Arkule, 1985; "Occupational Therapy", 1917; Quiroga, 1995; Upham, 1917). That is, our uniqueness has been in (a) the use of occupation as a curative or restorative force (the means), and (b) the view that enhanced occupational performance is the desired goal of therapy (the end).

Yet, as I have talked with occupational therapists in North America, Europe, and other world regions, I have been confronted with an apparent paradox — occupational therapists who know, implicitly, that they possess unique and important expertise, but who have difficulty articulating their uniqueness. Moreover, they often use evaluation and intervention methods that are so similar to those of their colleagues in such professions as physical therapy, neuropsychology, education, social work, and nursing, that any distinctions between occupational therapy and these professions become blurred and even abolished. As a result, ***our unique focus on occupation is not always obvious in practice***.

2.1 Common Intervention Methods

To clarify what I mean, I will describe the intervention methods I have observed occupational therapists use in their everyday practices. The focal point here will be the characteristics of the types of activities used as therapeutic media in occupational therapy settings — ***the things occupational therapists have their clients do as part of the client's therapy***.

As I use the term *activity* in this context, therefore, it should not be confused with the World Health Organization's (WHO, 2001) use of the terms *activity* and/or *participation* in the *International Classification of Functioning, Disability and Health* (ICF). Within ICF, both activity and participation can be viewed as occupation, as ***both involve engagement in active doing on the part of the person***. More specifically, in the ICF, the term *activity* is used to refer the "execution of a task or action by an individual" (WHO, p. 123). Thus, activity pertains to "doing" at the more discrete level of actions (e.g., performance skills, the smallest observable units of occupation) as well as at the more global level of the overall, task performance.[8] *Participation* refers to the person's involvement in life situations, from a more societal perspective, and within the naturalistic context of the person's daily life (WHO) (see the Appendix, Table 10 and Fisher, 2006b for more detail). In this chapter, I use the term *activity* to refer to both being engaged in doing (meaningful and purposeful activity, occupation) as well as "just doing" (activity without engagement as it is lacking in meaning and purpose from the perspective of the person). ***Unfortunately, not all of the activities used by occupational therapists involve engagement in occupation.***

2.1.1 Four Continua for Evaluating Activities Used as Intervention

As I proceed to introduce a broad method for categorizing the general types of activities that we can observe in occupational therapy practice settings, the astute reader will no doubt think of activities that do not fall neatly within one of these groups. It may help, therefore, to begin by thinking of four continua (see Figure 6).

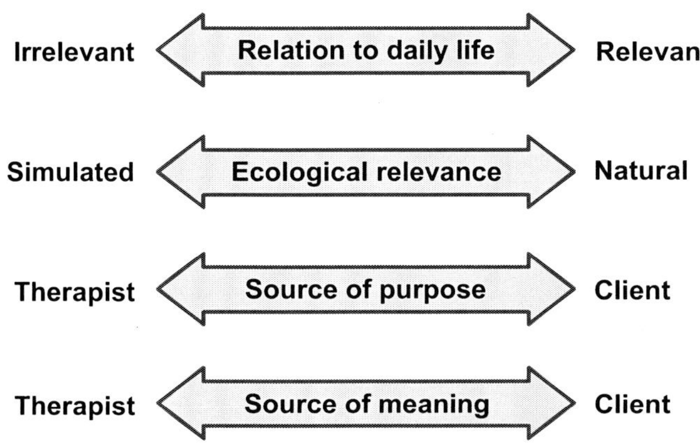

Figure 6. **Four continua that can be used to evaluate the characteristics of activities observed in occupational therapy practice settings.**

[8] Note that ICF uses *task* as a term to refer to a type of activity, and in so doing, uses the term *task* to refer to large units of action or "doing" (e.g., task performance), rather than to what it is the person will do or has done.

The first continuum indicates that an activity may be more or less ***relevant to daily life***. For example, dressing is relevant to daily life; whereas, placing pegs in a pegboard is generally irrelevant to daily life. Obviously, ***if our plan is for the client to be engaged in occupation, it is important that the activity be as relevant to daily life as possible***. To clarify further, within the context of these four continua, ***the first continuum is not intended to indicate that the activity is necessarily relevant to the particular person who is observed***. Relevance means only that the activity is related to daily life; to be relevant to a particular person, the activity must also be perceived by the person as having meaning and purpose within the context of his or her daily life. Meaning and purpose are the focus of the third and fourth continua in Figure 6, not this one.

The second continuum pertains to the ***ecological relevance*** of the activity. The activity may be more simulated or the activity may be more naturalistic. Simulated activities have one or more components that are contrived, artificial, or associated with a form of pretending that is not typically inherent to the activity. While simulated activities are not fully real, they should not be confused with play activities in which pretending is an important and integral aspect of the activity if the activity is "really" play. Ideally, the ***activities we observe in occupational therapy should occur in natural environments and involve using tools and materials that are typical for that daily life task***. When this occurs, the activities are ecologically relevant. For example, if a client is engaged in cooking activities in a kitchen located within a rehabilitation facility, that activity can be considered to be ecologically relevant. Of course, the ideal kitchen is the client's own kitchen. But if the hospital kitchen reasonably approximates a kitchen one might find in a home setting, the cooking activity performed there is still ecologically relevant.

The third and fourth continua indicate that the ***purpose*** and the ***meaning*** of the activity, respectively, may be generated more by the occupational therapist or generated more from within the client. That is, when the occupational therapist decides that a person would benefit by performing a task in order to attain a goal, the purpose and meaning come from the occupational therapist. It does not matter if the occupational therapist decides for the person that he or she should work on dressing skills, or that the client should put pegs into a pegboard so as to improve eye-hand coordination, the decision was made by the occupational therapist. In contrast, ***when the person has the opportunity to engage in a collaborative process with the occupational therapist as they jointly determine which activities might be most therapeutic, the person has the***

opportunity to choose activities that he or she perceives as having purpose and meaning in his or her life.

These four continua can be used to evaluate the characteristics of any activity we might observe and/or consider as intervention. The reader should not feel compelled to think in terms of "either/or" with respect to the anchor descriptors at either end of each continuum. Rather, my use of continua is to emphasize the idea that ***there are gradations as to the relative degree to which an activity meets any of these criteria. Ideally, any activity used as occupational therapy intervention will be offered as occupation***. This means that the activity is relevant to life and naturalistic. And, if it is indeed occupation, then the meaning and the purpose should be generated as much from within the client as is possible, given the client's performance limitations, level of motivation, and degree of self-awareness. That is, our goal in occupational therapy is to engage our clients in therapeutic occupation.

When I raise this point, the most common concern raised by occupational therapists concerns those clients "who do not want to do anything," "who do not know what they 'really' need," or "want me to decide what they should do." We much judge such comments with discernment, and our discernment must be guided by two overarching precautions:

1. ***We must always keep in mind that it is our ethical responsibility to (a) work in a manner that is client-centered and promotes the engagement of the client in the decision-making process, and (b) make every attempt to engage the client in activity that the client perceives as having meaning and/or purpose (i.e., occupation).***

2. ***We must carefully avoid choosing activities for our clients because (a) we think they are the ones in which our clients need to engage, and/or (b) someone else who is not part of the client constellation judges that the client needs to engage in them.***

2.1.2 Three Foci of Intervention

Another way to think about the activities used as therapy by occupational therapists is to consider the focus of the intervention. As shown in Figure 7, the focus of the intervention may be (a) compensation for lack of occupational skill; (b) reacquisition, development, or maintenance of occupational skill; or (c) restoration, development, or maintenance of person factors or body functions. Determining whether or not the activity is used in occupational therapy for purposes of compensation, acquisition, or restoration encourages the occupational therapist to make explicit his or her professional reasoning with regard to the intended purpose of the interventions. ***All three are appropriate foci for occupational therapy interventions.***

2.1.3 Six Types of Activities Used as Intervention by Occupational Therapists

As I now proceed to describe each of the six major activity groups, certain key characteristics of the activities will move from left to right along one or more of the four continua shown in Figure 6. I encourage occupational therapists to use these continua, the key foci represented in Figure 7, and the following broadly-defined activity groups as a ***basis for evaluating the activities they are using in practice in terms of their appropriateness as occupational therapy interventions.***

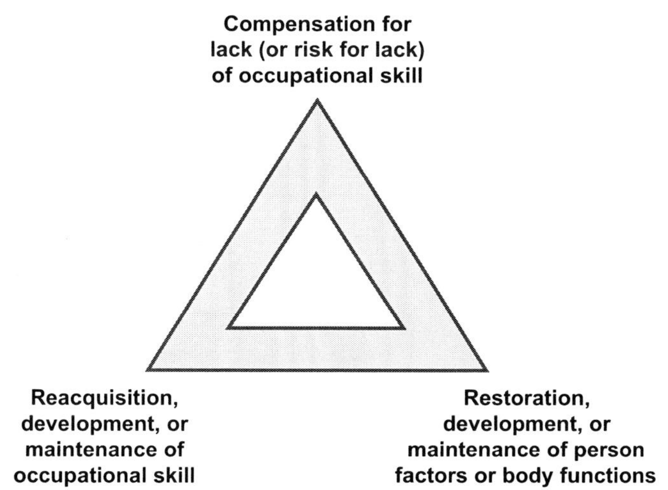

Figure 7. **Focus of occupation-based activities used in occupational therapy.**

Preparation

The first group of activities I have termed *preparation.* Examples of preparation activitics includc physical agent modalities (e.g., applications of heat, cold, transcutaneous electrical nerve stimulation, ultrasound), massage, and myofacial release. While the use of such approaches within occupational therapy is becoming more and more common (Bracciano, 2008), it is my view that they generally are most appropriately applied by other professionals. Passive range of motion exercises and applications of sensory stimulation, including (a) deep touch-pressure applied via the occupational therapist's hand or a brush, or (b) spinning a client in a net hammock (in the absence of active movement by the client or the client's engagement in activity).are also examples of preparation activities. Among the forms of preparation activities that are perhaps the most "traditional" within occupational therapy are positioning techniques associated with splinting or adapted seating.

The most readily apparent feature of preparation activities is that the client is a ***passive recipient*** of our interventions. From the perspective of the client, therefore, we cannot consider preparation "activities" to be activity at all because it is most often the case that the client is not doing anything and there is no client action to observe.

As we consider the four continua in Figure 6 in relation to preparation activities, we can recognize that they commonly lack relevance to daily life and they are rarely ecologically relevant. Moreover, because it is the occupational therapist who does the activity, the activity typically has no meaning or purpose to the client beyond that which has been understood by the client after the therapeutic purpose of the activity has been explained to the client by the occupational therapist.

When we consider Figure 7, it becomes clear that the focus of the preparation activity is on restoration, specifically the remediation of impairments or the restoration or development of body functions. Sometimes, they are even a pre-restorative activities performed by the occupational therapist in preparation for the client's later participation in some other form of therapeutic activity.

Rote Practice/Exercise

The second group of activities I have termed *rote practice/exercise*. Examples of rote practice/exercise include having the client use both hands to draw concentric circles on a blackboard to develop bilateral coordination, stretch Thera-Band®[9] or lift weights to improve strength, or stack cones to improve reaching capacity. Home exercise programs are often just that, forms of rote practice/exercise. Rote practice/exercise also includes cognitive-perceptual retraining activities (including cognitive retraining exercises performed using a computer) and cognitive-behavioral activities designed to improve insight or social awareness.

---

[9] Thera-Band Products, The Hygenic Corporation, 1245 Home Avenue, Akron, Ohio, USA, 44310.

The most salient feature of this type of activity is the therapeutic use of repetitive (rote) practice or exercise in order to develop, restore, or maintain body functions. As we consider the four continua in Figure 6, we can see that most rote practice/exercise activities have little or no relevance to daily life, and even when performed with real objects (e.g., chalk and a blackboard, computer), the fact that they involve repetitive practice out of the context of the performance of a real or simulated daily life task means that their ecological relevance is simulated rather than natural. The activity may have a purpose or goal, but more often than not, the purpose originated with the occupational therapist and not the client. In all probability, therefore, rote practice/exercise has little or no meaning to the client beyond that which is derived from the occupational therapist's explanation of the therapeutic purpose of the activity or the client's belief that performing exercises is "real therapy." ***When a client believes that "exercise is real therapy," the concepts of meaning and purpose become distorted and/or contrived because the meaning and purpose have come from bottom up reasoning and beliefs that are deeply imbedded in western cultures***; they are not originating from the client's perceptions of what daily life tasks the client needs or wants to be able to perform for purposes of assuming desired life roles and level of participation in society. Finally, when we evaluate rote practice/exercise activities in relation to Figure 7, we can see that the focus of the rote practice/exercise is on the restoration, development, or maintenance of person factors and body functions.

Simulated Occupation

The third group of activities I have termed *simulated occupation.* Simulated occupation includes any activity in which the purpose and/or the task tools and materials are simulated, contrived, artificial, or involve an element of pretending that is not natural to the task, but ***the occupational therapist attempts to approximate a daily life task performance***.

One type of simulated occupation involves the occupational therapist embedding rote practice or exercise in an activity in which some of the task objects and any potential meanings or purposes are contrived. For example, having a child cut modeling clay with a knife and fork or scoop beans with a spoon, telling him that he should pretend that he is eating, in as activity where some of the task objects as well as the purposes and meanings are contrived. Likewise, having a client place cones on a shelf and pretend that they are glasses and that he is putting the dishes away is a form of rote practice/exercise embedded in a simulated daily life task. The key elements are (a) that the cones have little relevance to the actual task being simulated; and (b) the occupational therapist contrived the "real life" purpose and meaning of the task for the client.

In other instances, the objects are real and not simulated, but some component of the task remains contrived. One example would be for an occupational therapist to tell a woman, "It is important for you to practice using your reacher. Let's imagine you need to throw away your used tissues," and then ask her to remove a number of tissues from a box of tissues and place them in a nearby wastebasket. While the activity attempts to approximate real life, and the reacher and tissues are real, the occupational therapist contrived the activity and specified its purpose.

Having a child pound nails into a board, encouraging him to pretend he is going to build a birdhouse is another example. Again, the objects are real and relevant to the occupational therapist-specified purpose, but there is to be no real birdhouse. Other examples include an occupational therapist having a child repetitively write one or more letters of the alphabet to develop fine motor coordination, or having an adult repetitively button buttons to restore buttoning skill. These activities remain simulated occupation because they are performed out of the context of real, naturalistic daily life task performances (e.g., writing a sentence to describe a picture drawn in the context of a teacher-specified schoolwork task, buttoning one's shirt in the context of getting dressed). In all of these examples, the purpose and the meaning have been contrived; they are more those of the occupational therapist than they are those of the clients.

As can be seen by all of the examples above, simulated occupation varies in the degree of simulation or the extent to which they are real. ***At their best, the occupational therapist makes every attempt to approximate real daily life tasks that have purpose and meaning to the client.*** Role play, a simulated occupation, often falls at the more natural end of the second continuum. For example, a group of young adults may choose to role play a job interview or ordering food at a local restaurant in preparation for engagement in the actual, naturalistic activity. In situations where the clients are not yet ready, are too fearful, or are unable to engage in the real activity (e.g., clients in locked units unable to go out into the community), such simulated occupation may be the "best possible alternative" to engagement in real occupation. ***At their worst***, however, as in the examples of practicing eating with clay or beans, or putting away cone "dishes," ***the occupational therapist merely embeds rote practice/exercise in activities the occupational therapist has contrived.*** If we examine the various examples I have provided above in relation to Figure 7, it should readily become apparent that simulated occupation can be focused on the restoration, development, or maintenance of body functions or person factors; or it can be focused on the reacquisition, development, or maintenance of occupational skill.

Differentiating between Rote Practice/Exercise and Simulated Occupation

The distinction between rote practice/exercise and simulated occupation focused on restoration can be subtle. For example, imagine a client who has been asked by the occupational therapist to sit on a mat table with her body weight partially supported on her extended hemiplegic right arm. The occupational therapist then asks her to use her left hand to pick up pegs from a bowl the occupational therapist has placed on the mat table to the client's left and to place the pegs in a solitaire game pegboard the occupational therapist has placed on the client's right side. Is this an example of rote practice/exercise or simulated occupation? If the woman is merely to place the pegs in the pegboard as a means of encouraging her to make postural adjustments to develop better postural control, then we can clearly consider this activity to be form of rote practice/exercise. If, however, the client is playing the game of solitaire, then it becomes simulated occupation — it is not natural to play solitaire in this manner, whether or not the client has any personal interest in playing solitaire.

As we reflect on the four continua in Figure 6 and continue to compare rote practice/exercise and simulated occupation, we can see that the daily life pertinence and ecological relevance likely is generally greater with simulated occupation than it is for rote practice/exercise, but because aspects of the activity are simulated, the daily life and ecological relevance remain limited. Unlike rote practice/exercise, where the meaning and purpose most often originate with the occupational therapist and not the client, the source of the meaning and purpose varies with simulated occupation. That is, when simulated occupation is at its best, it closely approximates a real life task performance that has meaning and purpose to the client. When, however, the purpose originates with the occupational therapist, the meaningfulness of the activity to the client also remains minimal. Finally, unlike rote practice/exercise, the focus of simulated occupation is not only on the remediation of underlying impairments, or restoration, development, or maintenance of body functions; it also can be on the reacquisition, development, or maintenance of occupational skill (see Figure 7).

Restorative Occupation

The fourth group of activities I have termed *restorative occupation*. As suggested by the name, the focus of restorative occupation is on the remediation of underlying impairments, or the restoration, development, or maintenance of person factors and body functions (see Figure 7). I have chosen to use the term *restorative*, but in doing so, I want to stress that I use it to refer to activities and models of practice that are used to (a) ***remediate*** underlying impairments and/or ***restore*** person factors and body functions that have been lost due to disease or injury, (b) ***develop*** person factors and body functions in persons who have not yet achieved age-appropriate occupational performance, or (c) ***maintain*** or ***enhance*** person factors or body functions in persons who currently perform daily life tasks very near or at a level that is expected for one's age. The latter includes the use of restorative occupation in the promotion of ***wellness*** and/or the ***prevention*** of functional decline (including ***maintenance*** of current level of performance) in persons who are at risk for loss of occupational performance.[10]

A critical characteristic of restorative occupation is that the client actively participates in occupation. This means that they are activities the ***client identifies*** as purposeful and meaningful. And, to the greatest extent possible, the occupational performance is relevant to daily life and naturalistic. The client performs daily life relevant activities using real objects, in natural environments. Therefore, as we consider Figure 6, a defining characteristic of restorative occupation is that it is located at or near the right end of each of the four continua.

An example of restorative occupation would be to use ***graded occupation*** (i.e., progressively grading the task challenge via modifying or adapting the task) to treat impairments of balance or reach. For example, imagine a client who loves to read. She has expressed concern that she is experiencing difficulty maintaining her balance while reaching for objects, including books, from shelves. Together, the client and the occupational therapist decide to go to her den and work on her problem areas. By progressively grading the task in terms of the challenges to her balance or the extent of reach required, engagement in an activity that has purpose and meaning to the client can be used for the remediation of her underlying impairments that are limiting her occupational performance. As her underlying abilities improve, she can begin to retrieve or return books that are heavier and heavier to progressively higher shelves.

---

[10] Both the terms *remediation* and *restoration* are used to label models of practice developed to remediate impairments and/or restore body function limitations (with a secondary goal of improving occupational performance). The term *remediation* is often perceived as having the more negative connotation due to its association with reductionistic, bottom–up models (e.g., medical model). While less negative, the term *restorative* still implies that the focus of such models is on the client's regaining lost body functions. As a result, my use of the term *restoration* does not overtly acknowledge our important role in habilitation and wellness. As I have sought a better term to refer to the models of practice in question, however, I have been unable to find a term that would be commonly understood among occupational therapists.

In another example of restorative occupation, the occupational therapist might attempt to remediate attentional deficits as the person engages in a favored card game. Progressively graded verbal cueing, or other forms of task gradations designed to promote the desired responses, enhance the therapeutic benefits of the intervention. The goal is the development or restoration of attentional mechanisms needed for "typical" occupational performances.

Differentiating between Simulated Occupation and Restorative Occupation

The distinction between better forms of simulated occupation focused on restoration and restorative occupation also can be subtle. The following case example of a man who had sustained a hand injury, shared with me by a colleague in Sweden, provides us with an excellent example of how we can think about the differences between the two types of activity.

When the occupational therapist asked her client about his interests, he stated that one of his favorite occupations and area of concern was rock climbing. The primary cause of his problems of occupational performance was that he lacked the muscle strength in his fingers needed to perform this, and other, favored occupations. Her initial reaction was to think that she could not engage him in rock climbing to develop muscle strength because of the lack of availability of a rock to climb (perhaps she also was thinking that she did not have the skills herself needed to rock climb). She then realized that there was a climbing wall in the gym of the occupational and physical therapy school adjacent to the outpatient clinic where she was working. She and her client were able to go to the gym and work on his developing hand strength in the context of climbing.

If we now consider this case example in terms of the second of the four continua in Figure 6, we can see how simulated occupation differs from restorative occupation. The key question to answer is: Is this rock climbing activity simulated occupation or is it restorative occupation? A climbing wall is not a rock, so perhaps it is a bit contrived. But the final determination of that will come from the client. Does he commonly practice on a climbing wall, or is it only "real" (natural) when he is up in the mountains climbing granite cliffs? If it is only real when he is up in the mountains, then we would consider this to be an example of simulated restorative occupation as we would position this activity on the second continuum somewhere beyond the middle point, but toward the right end. Climbing certainly is far less contrived than it would have been if she had him perform finger strengthening exercises using putty or a rubber ball (rote practice/exercise). If, however, he commonly practices on a climbing wall (a real, routine occupation), then we can judge it to be restorative occupation because it is naturalistic and contextual, given that practicing on a climbing wall in a gym is a typical physical environment in which he would practice rock climbing. That is, we would place the activity at the far right end of the continuum.

Acquisitional Occupation

The fifth group of activities I have termed *acquisitional occupation*. The direct aim of acquisitional occupation is to enable the client to reacquire, develop, or maintain effective actions so that the client can perform daily life tasks in a manner that is typical for persons of the same age, gender, and cultural group. Just as with restorative occupation, the client actively participates in occupation, activities which are relevant to daily life and naturalistic, and the client identifies as purposeful and meaningful. This means that a defining characteristic of acquisitional occupation is that it is located at or near the right end of each of the four continua shown in Figure 6. In fact, ***the only difference between acquisitional occupation and restorative occupation is that the focus of acquisitional occupation is on the reacquisition, development, or maintenance of occupational skill rather than restoration, development, or maintenance of person factors or body functions*** (see Figure 7). Moreover, in a manner similar to restorative occupation and restorative models of practice, acquisitional occupation and acquisitional models of practice can be applied for purposes of (a) ***reacquiring*** occupational performance skills in persons who have lost them, (b) ***developing*** occupational performance skills in persons who have not yet achieved age-appropriate occupational performance, or (c) ***maintaining*** or ***enhancing*** occupational performance skills in persons who currently perform daily life tasks near or at a level that is expected for one's age and who are at risk for loss of occupational performance.[11]

Typical examples of acquisitional occupation would be for the occupational therapist to work with a client group of adolescents to improve their social interaction skills while they socially interact in the context of making a cake for one of their mothers, or to use grocery shopping as a therapeutic occupation for a man who wants to be able to shop for food for his family. In both cases, the occupational therapist

---

[11] ***Wellness***, ***prevention***, and ***maintenance*** can ultimately be viewed as the same thing as all three are based on the idea of "building up" (i.e., enhancing) a person's quality of occupational performance to counteract any declines that might occur.

progressively grades the task challenge as the client's level of occupational skill improves. The focus of the intervention involves the person or others in the client constellation ***engaging in the performance of progressively graded tasks so as to improve their performances of the same or very similar tasks***. In all cases, the tasks performed are ones that the client needs and wants to perform and has prioritized as targets for intervention.

Comparing Acquisitional Occupation and Restorative Occupation

Restorative occupation and acquisitional occupation share many features in common. That is, both involve collaborative consultation and education, and the use of progressive grading of the task (via modifying or adapting). Moreover, both can be implemented as direct intervention or as indirect intervention (see Figure 8).

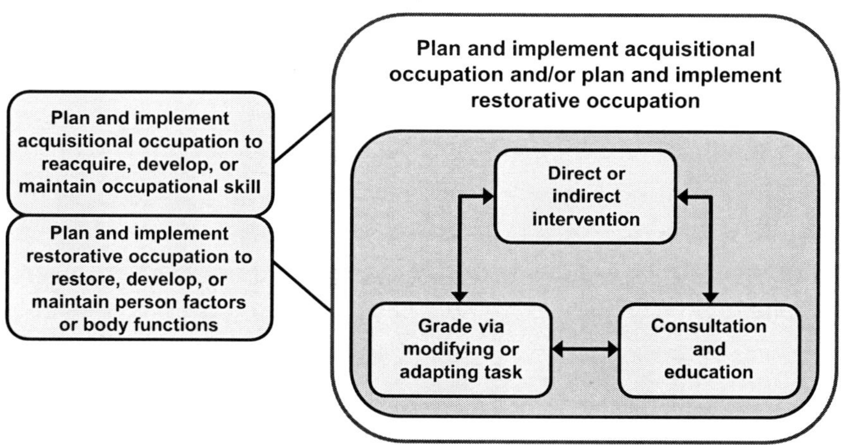

Figure 8. **Schematic representation of acquisitional and restorative occupation.**

As is discussed in more detail in Chapter 3, ***collaborative consultation*** pertains to collaborating with the client to (a) identify which task performances are to be prioritized as targets of intervention, (b) determine the client's desired outcomes (i.e., goals), and (c) choose what interventions will be implemented and how they will be implemented. The use of ***grading*** (via modifying or adapting the task) is used for purposes of altering the task challenge to meet the baseline ability of the client, and then gradually increasing the challenge as the client's quality of performance improves. ***Educational principles*** are used in the process of teaching a client and the client's learning, through practice. When educational principles are applied in the context of restorative occupation, the focus is on the client learning underlying capacities (e.g., improved motor control, improved insight and awareness, use of cognitive-behavioral techniques to reduce stress or pain). When educational principles are applied in the context of acquisitional occupation, the focus is directly on occupational skills and quality of daily life task performance (e.g., improved dressing skill, improved social interaction skill). Finally, when it is ***direct intervention***, the occupational therapist works directly with the client. It becomes ***indirect intervention*** when the occupational therapist teaches someone else (e.g., parent, teacher, aide) to implement the occupation-based intervention.

Thus, to the casual observer, the focus of the intervention may not be apparent. In both cases, what is observed is the client's engagement in occupation, and the focus of the intervention involves the client engaging in the performance of progressively graded tasks so as to improve performance of the same or similar tasks. In all cases, the tasks performed are ones that the client prioritized as a target for intervention because they were ones that the person or others in the client constellation needed and wanted to be able to perform.

The difference between acquisitional occupation and restorative occupation lies primarily in the professional reasoning of the occupational therapist. Often, it is only through discussion with the occupational therapist that the actual focus becomes clear. For example, I recently observed an occupational therapist who was working with a group of persons with psychiatric disorders (i.e., a client group). The client group was engaged in a social activity that involved group planning of an outing; they were to decide when and where they would go. The occupational therapist sat with the group, and, as needed, provided cues to facilitate social interaction. I assumed, therefore, that the focus of the group activity was acquisitional — to promote social interaction skills. Contrary to my expectations, when I later interviewed the occupational therapist, I learned that she had used the group activity to promote awareness of their disabilities. Thus, for the occupational therapist, the focus of the group activity was restorative — to develop an underlying body function, insight.

Adaptive Occupation

The final group of activities I have termed *adaptive occupation.* As with restorative or acquisitional occupation, a critical characteristic is the client's active participation in occupations that are chosen by the client. The activities, therefore, are relevant to daily life, naturalistic, and purposeful and meaningful to the client (see Figure 6). In fact, the only distinction between adaptive occupation and restorative or acquisitional occupation is that ***adaptive occupation is focused directly on compensation for ineffective occupational skill and not restoration, development, or maintenance of person factors and body functions, or the reacquisition, development, or maintenance of occupational skill*** (see Figure 7). When a person uses assistive devices, receives help from another, or performs daily life tasks in an alternative manner so as to overcome or compensate for ineffective actions, the person is engaging in adaptive occupation (see Figure 9). The intent is to ***enable the client to perform activities in a new way that is somehow different from how people would typically perform the task***.

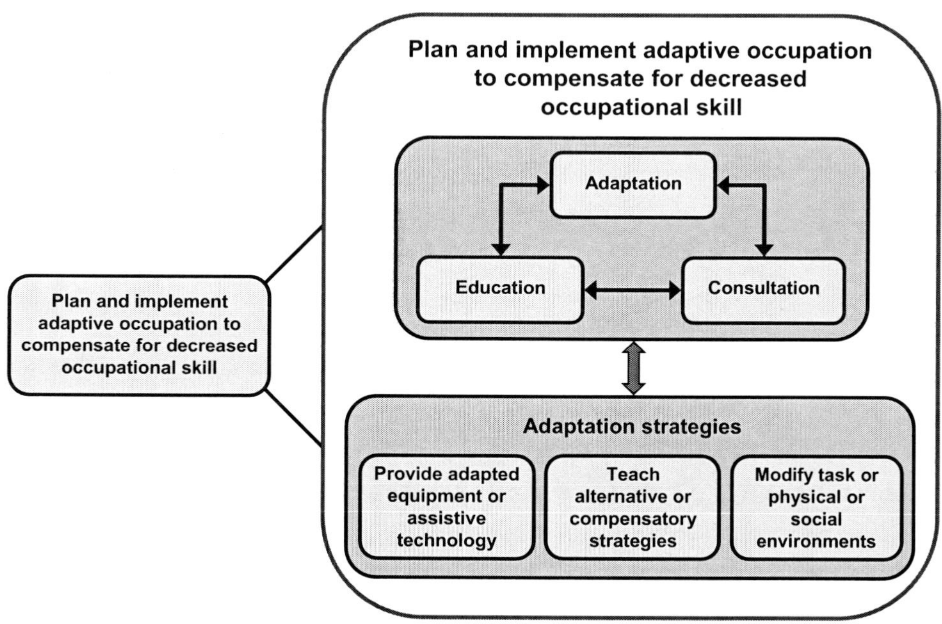

Figure 9. Schematic representation of adaptive occupation.

More specifically, when the focus of the intervention is on *compensation*, there is acknowledgement that the reacquisition or development of effective actions needed for "typical performance" is currently not a realistic goal (i.e., indirectly via restorative occupation, or directly via acquisitional occupation). The direct aim, therefore, is to introduce adaptations to compensate for decreased occupational skill. In such situations, ***the expectation is that the person will perform his or her daily life tasks in a manner that is somehow different*** from what would be considered typical. Using a reacher to pick up one's socks from the floor (adapted device), tying one's shoes with one hand (alternative or compensatory technique), or getting dressed with verbal cues or the physical assistance of a caregiver (modify social environment) are ***not*** typical ways for a young adult to get dressed.

An example of adaptive occupation might involve engaging a client with low endurance in a desired laundry task. While she is doing the family laundry, the occupational therapist would use education to teach her alternative ways to manage her carrying the laundry to and from the laundry area, load and unload the washer and dryer, and so on. One strategy might be to teach her to do smaller loads of laundry more often so that there would be only a limited number of items in each family member's laundry basket. Another might be to teach her to use a cart to transport the laundry to the laundry area.

The key characteristic of adaptive occupation is the use of adaptation to alter or change the activity so that the client can perform it successfully (Mosey, 1986), although the ***method used is no longer typical***. While the goal of adaptive occupation is not to improve the woman's endurance, it is possible, that her endurance will eventually improve secondarily to her enhanced engagement in occupation.

It is also important to keep in mind that ***consultation and education*** are also important components of adaptive occupation (see Figure 9). In the example above, the occupational therapist already had developed a collaborative consultative relationship with the woman with low endurance. Moreover, before she actually implemented adaptive occupation, the occupational therapist realized that it was important for her to extend the consultative partnerships to include the family members who would be impacted by the implemented adaptations and include them in the process of designing and implementing any suggested adaptations. When they became involved in the process, they suggested that they carry their own laundry baskets to and from the laundry area. Obviously, minimal education was needed. In other instances, the educational component will be more extensive (e.g., teaching a caregiver to transfer a person who has sustained a stroke to and from the toilet and/or bathtub, and providing opportunities for the caregiver to practice and learn to safely transfer the person).

Differentiating between Acquisitional or Restorative Occupation and Adaptive Occupation

Just as the distinction between acquisitional and restorative occupation is typically made based on the occupational therapist's professional reasoning, the ***distinction between acquisitional or restorative occupation and adaptive occupation often is made based on the professional reasoning of the occupational therapist*** as to what he or she views as the primary goal of the intervention. The distinction is clarified by answering the question: Is the activity adapted to allow the client's engagement at a modified level over an extended period of time (adaptive occupation; compensation for decreased occupational skill), or are the adaptations gradually changing gradations in task challenge that are progressively removed as person factors, body functions, or occupational skills improve (restorative or acquisitional occupation, respectively)? The woman who now uses her cart to transport her laundry has learned a new way of doing, and she will continue to use this new, adapted method for some time. In contrast, the woman who loves to read discussed earlier intends to gather and replace her books in a typical manner as soon as she is stronger. In the former case, the adaptation is intended to be relatively permanent. In the latter case, the task gradations are dynamically changed as the client improves during the course of therapy. Those gradations are implemented by progressively modifying or adapting the task challenge.

2.2 Legitimate Activities for Occupational Therapy

What then are the legitimate activities for occupational therapy?[12] Kielhofner (1997) has argued that the emerging paradigm of occupational therapy requires that we recognize occupation as the level of intervention. I believe this should be true whether the intervention involves (a) engaging the person in restorative occupation as a preliminary step toward enhanced occupational performance, (b) engaging the person in acquisitional occupation for purposes directly improving occupational skill and enhancing occupational performance; or (c) engaging the person in adaptive occupation to directly enhance occupational performance through compensation. Certainly, if we tie current practice to our philosophical base, then ***the clear emphasis of our***

[12] As noted in Chapter 1, my use of the term *legitimate activities* should not be confused with what Mosey (1986) refers to as the *legitimate tools* of occupational therapy.

interventions must be restorative, acquisitional, and adaptive occupation — only then are our interventions occupation-based.

My advocating for the use of restorative, acquisitional, and adaptive occupation is based on the premise that "occupation as not just any activity, not even just any purposeful activity, but . . . activity that is both meaningful and purposeful to the person who engages in it" (Fisher, 1998, p. 511). A critical characteristic of all three forms of occupation (i.e., restorative, acquisitional, adaptive) is that they are activities that are ***chosen*** by the client and that the ***client identifies*** as purposeful and meaningful. And, to the greatest extent possible, the occupational performance is ***naturalistic*** and ***contextual***. The client performs the activities using real objects, in natural environments.

I also believe there is ***some justification for the occasional use of simulated occupation***, especially with clients who lack motivation, self-awareness, or are too fearful to engage in activities that we might feel are more relevant to their daily life needs. In this case, simulated activities or role play may be used early in the intervention in an attempt to facilitate the client's active participation and to increase motivation and/or self-confidence. If the person (or others in the client constellation) lacks motivation, is unwilling, or is unable to perform the task him- or herself, the occupational therapist may need to choose an activity for the client based on his or her best judgment about what activities will have potential to have meaning and purpose for the client. As a result, the client may initially "go through the motions" of implementing the task performance, but the person's sense of purpose and meaning in relation to the activity likely will be minimal. The hope is that purpose and meaning will emerge. ***If such activities have no apparent therapeutic benefit, and/or the client remains unwilling to engage in occupation, then perhaps we should turn the intervention over to other professionals whose methods and focus may be more appropriate.***

In other instances where simulated occupation is justified, the client may be motivated to engage in meaningful and chosen occupations, but for some reason cannot. While the activities remain somewhat contrived, ideally our clients become involved in choosing the simulated activities they view as relevant to their lives (e.g., role play in preparation for actual engagement in a desired outing to a restaurant). ***Whenever we choose to use simulated occupation, we must keep in mind the evidence that such methods are not always as effective as is performance of real tasks, using real objects, in natural contexts*** (cf. Ma, Trombly, & Robinson-Podolski, 1999; Mathiowetz & Wade, 1995; Wu, Trombly, Lin, & Tickle-Degnan, 2000).

The preparation activities of splinting and adaptive seating have traditionally been viewed as legitimate methods for occupational therapy. Otherwise, preparation and rote practice/exercise are rarely justified. We must not, therefore, be too quick to rationalize our use of preparation and rote practice/exercise rather than ***acknowledge professional boundaries and the reality that there are other professionals whose expertise is greater and more relevant to the client's needs***. We also must be willing to question the validity of the view that an appropriate occupational therapy intervention program often involves progressing a client from preparation or rote practice/exercise to occupation, either within or between intervention sessions.

We do not like to think that what we are doing is not legitimate occupational therapy. But, whether we want to admit it to ourselves or not, there are still many occupational therapists in the United States, Europe, and other world regions who continue to ***emphasize*** the use of preparation and rote practice/exercise for the remediation of underlying impairments and the restoration or development of person factors and body functions, justifying their programs to themselves and others by stating that their ***ultimate*** goal is improved occupational performance. Still others often use simulated occupation, even when engagement of a client in occupation is possible, justifying their use of simulated occupation based on time, space, or other demands within their work settings. Each of us is, therefore, challenged to ask three very important questions.

1. ***If I examine the activities I currently am using with my clients, is a significant proportion of time devoted to activities best defined as preparation, rote practice/exercise, or simulated occupation, or is the greatest proportion devoted to activities best defined as restorative, acquisitional, and adaptive occupation?***

   There is no magic rule here, but as a guideline, I recommend that no more than a small percentage of a client's occupational therapy intervention time be spent on preparation, rote practice/exercise, and/or simulated occupation. Moreover, preparation, rote practice/exercise, and/or simulated occupation should ***only*** be used with the small percentage of our clients who cannot or will not participate in restorative, acquisitional, or adaptive occupation. Finally, simulated occupation, when it is well designed, focused on the client's needs and desires, and as natural as possible, is always preferred over preparation or rote practice.

2. ***As I look around my occupational therapy work environment, do I see the objects of occupation arranged in natural contexts, or do I see weights, cones,***

pegboards, physical agent modalities, mat tables, bolsters, or other objects that have no meaning or purpose to my clients?

As Lindstrom and Westropp (1999) so clearly articulated, the physical layout of our clinic spaces can be a major impediment to our use of restorative, acquisitional, and adaptive occupation. When they examined their own clinic, they found that

> *First, the basic physical layout of the clinic was an impediment. The tools that are generally considered most conductive [sic] to providing opportunities for meaningful occupation (e.g., hand tools, horticultural supplies, cutlery, manicure kits) were locked in cabinets and closets. . . .*
>
> *Second, supplies to support occupation-based treatment were "invisible." Contrived activities, such as range of motion arcs, resistive peg boards, and clothespins, were arranged on the counters within easiest reach. Evidence of rote exercise (pulleys, hand and wrist weights, weight dowels) was prominently displayed throughout the clinic. . . . No wonder it was easier to use cones.* (p. 2)

After they had reorganized their clinic spaces and increased their use of occupation-based group activities, Lindstrom and Westropp (1999) found that their interventions became more creative as well as more cost-effective, and that their clients became more engaged in their own intervention programs.

3. ***How are my evaluation methods and intervention programs different from those of physical therapists, neuropsychologists, and others?***

As we attempt to answer this question, we can think not only about the activities and tools we use, but also about the professional reasoning that underlies our interventions. Are we reasoning as an occupational therapist, or more like a physical therapist, art therapist, neuropsychologist, educator, or some other professional? All of these other professionals have as their ultimate goal improved functional performance; ***none of them focuses directly on occupation*** or the ability of their clients to engage in the process of performing those daily life tasks that the clients view as being meaningful, purposeful, and relevant to their daily lives.

3. ASSUMPTIONS ABOUT PEOPLE AND PRINCIPLES OF INTERVENTION

Each model of practice has incorporated into it theoretical assumptions that the occupational therapist makes when applying that model. These assumptions tell us about the occupational nature of people and how they change. They also tell us what therapeutic mechanisms effect those changes. The principles of intervention clarify the nature of interventions implemented using that model.

Embedded within the OTIPM is (a) an articulation of the compensatory model and (b) the assertion that occupational therapists make linkages to the many restorative and acquisitional models of practice available for our use. Any of these models, including the compensatory model, can be taught and used in isolation of the OTIPM.

Another assertion, however, is that their therapeutic applications within the OTIPM ensures the use of a professional reasoning process that guarantees they are implemented in a manner that is indeed truly top–down, client-centered, and occupation-based. That is, the advantage of applying restorative and acquisitional models in the context of the OTIPM is that they become occupational-therapy-specific applications of those models. Almost all restorative and acquisitional models (and their associated evaluation and intervention strategies) were developed for use outside our profession (e.g., biomechanical, behavioral, developmental, neurodevelopmental, humanistic).

The compensatory model presented in this chapter represents a new, expanded version of concepts originally articulated by Trombly (1995c). The theoretical assumptions and the principles of intervention are, therefore, presented here in full even though the compensatory model is a model in its own right. In contrast, the theoretical assumptions and the principles for intervention for restorative and acquisitional models presented here are intended to be generic and to compliment those articulated by the authors of the original models.

3.1 Theoretical Assumptions

The following theoretical assumptions apply to the OTIPM:

1. Occupational performance unfolds as a transaction between a person[13] and the environment as he or she enacts a task.
2. Occupational performance occurs within a client-centered context that provides the framework for understanding, evaluating, and interpreting the person's occupational performance.
3. The client-centered performance context is comprised of 10 interrelated dimensions — the environmental dimension, the role dimension, the motivational dimension, the task dimension, the cultural dimension, the social dimension, the societal dimension, the body function dimension, the temporal dimension, and the adaptation dimension.
4. The ability of a person to perform daily life tasks is influenced by each of the 10 dimensions of the client-centered performance context.
5. Loss of competence in occupational performance can occur as a result of a change or disruption in any of the 10 dimensions of the client-centered performance context, including a change in person factors and body functions, "loss of motivation, drastic changes in environment, or cultural inaccessibility" (Trombly, 1995d, p. 23). Occupational dysfunction also can occur when the individual fails to develop competence in occupational performance.
6. A sufficient level of motivational, as well as neuromuscular, biomechanical, cognitive, and psychosocial person factors and body functions are needed for both learning and for daily life task performance that is effortless, efficient, safe, independent, socially appropriate, and satisfying.
7. When a person lacks, or is at risk of losing, competence in occupational performance that person is viewed as a learner who needs to gain, regain, or maintain competence in occupational performance.
8. People can develop (via habilitation), reacquire or regain (via rehabilitation), or enhance and/or maintain (via wellness and/or prevention of decline) the ability to perform daily life tasks through participation in restorative, acquisitional, and/or adaptive occupation.
9. Occupation-based education programs can be used when the focus of the intervention is to provide education programs (via seminars, lectures, and workshops,) for large groups, and that are focused on discussion of their daily lives and related occupational performances.

[13] In this section, I use the term person to refer to human beings in general, whether or not that person has been referred for or seeks occupational therapy services, is a member of a client constellation, or is a member of a client group.

10. The primary goal of restorative occupation is the remediation of underlying impairments, or the restoration, development, or maintenance of person factors and body functions that underlie or are required for skilled occupational performance.
11. The primary goal of acquisitional occupation is the reacquisition, development, or maintenance of occupational skill in order to directly reacquire, develop, or maintain effective goal-directed actions of occupational performance.
12. The primary goal of adaptive occupation is to compensate for ineffective (or prevent decline of effective) goal-directed actions of occupational performance through the provision of adapted equipment or assistive technology, teaching the client to perform tasks using alternative or compensatory techniques, or modifying the task or the physical or social environments.
13. The primary goal of occupation-based education programs is to provide large groups opportunities to discuss possible intervention, wellness, and/or preventive strategies within a more classroom-like format. Rather than having the opportunity to practice and learn during the education program, the program may include information and discussion about strategies the persons are encouraged to try later, after completion of the education program.
14. When the person is unable to engage in restorative, acquisitional, and/or adaptive occupation, the ***temporary use*** of simulated occupation may be appropriate.
15. The primary goal of simulated occupation, like restorative or acquisitional occupation, may be the (a) remediation of underlying impairments; (b) restoration, development, or maintenance of person factors and body functions; or (c) reacquisition, development, or maintenance of occupational skill in order to directly or indirectly restore, develop, or maintain effective occupational performance.
16. When the person has persistent person factor and body function limitations that cannot be restored or developed through timely and cost-effective participation in restorative (or simulated) occupation, and/or the person is not able to reacquire or develop occupational skill through occupational skills training (given the time and resources available), the occupational therapist teaches the person to adapt his or her methods, tools, and environments to enable the ability to perform daily life tasks through compensation.
17. Whenever possible, the person with a persistent disability is viewed as one who can become an effective problem-solver, capable of learning, generalizing, and designing new adaptations as the need arises.

18. When the person with a persistent disability is unable to become an effective problem-solver or learn new adaptations, interventions should focus on those modifications to the physical and social environments needed to support the person's continued occupational performance.
19. When no adaptations can compensate for the person's residual disability, the person will need to eliminate the task from his or her daily life, manage the task by directing others, or accept the assistance of another person.
20. When caregiver training is provided as part of the intervention, the caregiver becomes the learner.

3.2 Principles of Intervention

In this section, I present general principles for intervention that apply to the entire occupational therapy intervention process. These ***general principles for intervention*** also clarify the relationship between the stages of the OTIPM and the components of what is often referred to as the occupational therapy process (e.g., referral, screening, assessment, goal-setting, intervention, reevaluation, discharge) (cf. the Appendix; Reed & Sanderson, 1999). This is followed by a presentation of ***specific principles related to the therapeutic use of adaptive, acquisitional, and restorative occupation, and occupation-based educational programs***.

3.2.1 General Principles

Whether the occupational therapist implements adaptive, acquisitional, or restorative occupation, and/or occupation-based educational programs, there are a number of general principles that are applicable to the provision of quality occupational therapy services. Among them are the following:

1. ***Develop therapeutic rapport and collaborative relationships***: Developing and maintaining a relationship of mutual confidence and respect between an occupational therapist and client is critical to the occupational therapy intervention process. Such a relationship requires an atmosphere where there is open sharing between equals — the occupational therapist and the client.[14] The occupational

[14] Again, as I use the term, the *client* may be a person who seeks/was referred for occupational therapy services, a client constellation (e.g., a person with a disability and his or her caregiver, members of his or her family, members of his or her educational team), or a client group (e.g., group of persons with brain injury, an organization comprised of administrators and a group of employees, a population of well older adults living in a large city), depending on toward whom our services are focused.

therapist brings to this collaborative (consultative) partnership expertise related to available intervention strategies and knowledge related to potential outcomes. The client brings expertise related to his or her values, interests, goals, and priorities. A potential threat to establishing such a partnership is our failing to let go of our own personal goals for the client, and listening instead to those of the client.

2. ***Carry out an initial evaluation***: The initial occupational therapy evaluation process involves establishing the client-centered performance context, identifying resources and limitations within that performance context, identifying the client's self-reported problems and priorities related to occupational performance, implementing performance analyses, defining and describing actions of performance that the client does and does not perform effectively, and defining/clarifying or interpreting the cause of those problems. In the case of wellness and prevention, the focus is often on any problems the client is at risk of developing in the future.

3. ***Document the results of the client's initial evaluation***: All documentation should follow a top–down, "occupation-first" progression. This means that a summary of (a) the client's background information (summary of the resources and limitations in the global client-centered performance context), (b) the reason for referral, (c) the client's reported problems and priorities related to occupational performance, (d) the client's ***global baseline*** level of observed occupational performance (using the six qualitative continua proposed in Chapter 6 — level of effort, degree of efficiency, degree of safety, level of need for assistance, degree of social appropriateness, and degree of satisfaction with occupational performance), (e) the client's ***specific baseline*** level of observed performance (the actions of performance that support and limit effective occupational performance), and (f) the cause or reasons for the client's diminished occupational performance (see the Appendix, Table 11 and Figure 18). The documentation of the client's observed baseline level of performance ***always*** precedes documentation of our interpretation of the cause of the client's limitations in occupational performance. ***Documenting an observable and measureable baseline level of observed occupational performance is the first step in effective documentation for use in program evaluation and evidence-based practice.*** Such baselines may also include level of self-reported satisfaction with occupational performance, degree of experienced pain during occupational performance, and the like.

4. ***Establish the expected outcomes and document the client's goals***: This step involves collaborating with the client to establish client-centered goals that represent the client's ***desired next level of occupational performance***. Because the *client* may be a person, others in the client constellation (e.g., a caregiver, a family member, an educational team), or a client group (including an organization comprised of administrators and/or a group of employees), as we collaborate with the client to establish client-centered goals, we often will do so with persons in addition to or other than the person who seeks/was referred for occupational therapy services. In this process, ***we must take extreme care not to impose our goals or those of others on the person who seeks/was referred for occupational therapy services***.

   As we document the client's goals, we again use the six qualitative continua proposed in Chapter 6. It is important to point out that ***we do not indicate in the client's goals what our methods of intervention will be*** (e.g., consultation, education, adaptive occupation). That is, we indicate what the client will do, not what the occupational therapist will do. Our methods of intervention, the general strategies discussed below, will be documented later, in the intervention plan.

   It is also important to consider that while we may choose to include in the goal the expected adaptive equipment (e.g., wheelchair, grab bars, over-edge bath bench) and/or strategies the client will use, as they may be viewed as a condition of the client's performance, doing so can have an important disadvantage. For example, an occupational therapist may document the client's goal as: *Frank will stand at the sink and independently perform his morning grooming tasks (e.g., brushing teeth, shaving).* Should it become the case that Frank can independently manage grooming, but only when sitting, he will not have met his goal. If, however, his goal had been written as: *Frank will independently perform his morning grooming tasks (e.g., brushing teeth, shaving)*, then the occupational therapist and Frank would be free to collaborate in the process of determining which strategies are acceptable to Frank and which of those is most effective.

   Finally, if a client has sought/been referred for occupational therapy services that extend beyond an initial evaluation (e.g., evaluation and intervention, as needed), the client's goals are documented along with the results of the initial evaluation. This is true even if the client will be referred elsewhere for further occupational therapy services (see the Appendix, Table 11 and Figures 17 to 19). ***Documenting observable and measureable goals is the second critical step of***

effective documentation for use in program evaluation and evidence-based practice.

5. ***Determine therapeutic strategies and document the intervention plan***: These are general (global) strategies for implementing interventions — graded restorative or acquisitional occupation, consultation, education, as well as the adaptation strategies (i.e., provide adaptive equipment or assistive technology, teach alternative or compensatory techniques, or modify task or the physical or social environment) that the occupational therapist plans to use in the intervention process. These general strategies are documented in the intervention plan.

6. ***Develop mutually-agreed-upon interventions***: The specific interventions (e.g., provide the client with a reacher, engage client in a cooking group to enhance social skills) are those that are developed as the client and the occupational therapist work together in a collaborative partnership. This partnership is based on therapeutic rapport (Tickle-Degnen, 2008), and the specific interventions are based on the general therapeutic strategies documented in the intervention plan. These specific interventions are ***not*** usually documented as part of the intervention plan.

7. ***Implement principles of restorative, acquisitional, adaptive occupation, and/or occupation-based education programs***: These principles are listed in Sections 3.2.2 to 3.2.4 below.

8. ***Reevaluate to verify that the intervention was effective and document the outcome attained***: Reevaluation involves verification that the client has met the client's goals. Since occupational therapy goals pertain to enhanced and satisfying occupational performance, reevaluation includes, but is not limited to, implementing performance analyses of those task performances that were targeted in the client's original goals and redefining the actions of performance that the client does and does not perform effectively. Since enhanced occupational performance also includes improved client satisfaction, reevaluation may also involve assessment of changes in client satisfaction. ***Documenting the client's new baseline level of performance (reevaluation baseline), in a form that is measurable and observable, is the third critical step toward effective documentation for use in program evaluation and evidence-based practice.***

9. ***Document results of intervention***: Documentation of the results involves comparing the client's baseline level of performance to the client's goal and the outcome attained. This comparison enables the occupational therapist to judge whether or not the client met the goal or made progress toward the goal. Documentation of the result provides us with the evidence we need to communicate the importance of occupational therapy in enhancing the lives of our clients, as well as justifying payment of occupational therapy services by health care payers. ***Without the documentation of the client's baseline level of performance, goals, and outcomes of intervention, documentation of the result — change effected through occupational therapy interventions — cannot be achieved.***

10. ***Target new client priorities as they arise***: As the client makes changes in occupational performance, additional tasks may become priorities for intervention. The client's baseline level of performance, goals, expected outcomes, and general therapeutic strategies must be established for each of these new tasks and documented in the appropriate place (e.g., weekly progress note). After mutually-agreed-upon interventions are implemented and their effectiveness reevaluated, the effectiveness of those interventions also should be documented in ***progress notes*** or a ***discharge summary***.

    As noted above, all documentation should use occupation-first language, and follow a top–down progression, with occupational performance documented before underlying impairments or person factors and body functions. A recommended structure for documentation of an initial occupational therapy evaluation is shown in Table 1 (see also the Documentation Examples in Chapters 4 and 5, and the Appendix, Table 11 and Figures 17 to 19, for more information about and examples of documentation).

3.2.2 Principles of Adaptive Occupation

Collaborative Consultation

Collaborative consultation can be likened to therapeutic rapport in that it is based on a mutual and collaborative relationship among equals (Tickle-Degnen, 2008). An effective consultative process often requires that the occupational therapist enter into a shared partnership not only with the person and others in the client constellation, but also develop further consultative partnerships with others who may work with the client, but who are ***not*** part of the client constellation (e.g., caregivers, other professionals, service extenders — aides and assistants). The development of sound collaborative relationships is critical for ensuring that each member of the partnership can communicate the information necessary for shared problem-solving. The steps or principles of the collaborative consultative process are listed below.

Table 1 A Recommended Structure for Top–down and "Occupation-first" Documentation of an Initial Occupational Therapy Evaluation

- Background information (occupation-related/relevant history)
- Reason for referral to occupational therapy
- Reported level of occupational performance (strengths and problems of occupational performance, based on client report)
- Occupational priorities (prioritized task performances)
- Observed level of occupational performance (global and specific baseline quality of occupational performance)
- Interpretation of cause (person, body function, environmental, or societal factors that contribute to diminished occupational performance)
- Client's goals
- Intervention plan

1. ***Identify critical persons to include as members of the consultative partnership (e.g., therapist, client, caregiver, service extender, other professional)***: The consultative partnership always includes the person who seeks/was referred to occupational therapy and others in the client constellation. The consultative partnership often extends to also include persons who are not already part of the client constellation or involved in the intervention process. The members of the extended consultative partnership will be those persons who have access to needed information or skills, as well as those who will be impacted by the proposed changes. For example, members of the client's family[15] who are living with him or her, or who are the persons who will be providing the client with assistance, are important members of the consultative partnership. Family members and service

[15] I use the term *family* to refer to all members of a client's significant social group, which may include parents, children, spouses, partners, or friends.

providers not already in the client constellation who will be impacted by the intervention should be included in the extended consultative partnership. If they are not included in the intervention process, they may not accept or fully understand the reasons for any adaptations that are proposed. As a result, there is an increased risk that they may impede the success of the proposed interventions.

2. ***Establish collaborative relationships***: Building on the principles of therapeutic rapport (Tickle-Degnen, 2008), the occupational therapist establishes connection and open communication, and promotes an atmosphere of mutual and collaborative exchange among the members of the client constellation and the extended consultative partnership. The consultative process is maximized when ***openness and trust*** are fostered and all members feel free to voice concerns and offer potential solutions.

3. ***Determine which members are most appropriate to implement intervention — the recipient of the consultative process (caregiver, service extender, or other professional)***: As further collaborative relationships are established and adaptations proposed, the person(s) who will be responsible for implementing the adaptations will be identified. For example, the family (recipient) may need to hire someone to install grab bars in a bathroom or learn (via education) to effectively cue a client or set up the environment to promote the client's competence in occupational performance.

Adaptation

The successful application of adaptation is dependent on multiple factors, including the client's perception of the usefulness of the adaptation and the client's willingness to accept the need for adaptation. Effective adaptation, therefore, requires that we follow the principles originally proposed by Trombly (1995c). I have expanded them here based on my experience with the OTIPM.

1. ***Know principles and methods of adaptation***: These include methods for modifying physical and social environments (e.g., providing social supports and/or assistance, making physical modifications to the environment, changing the task complexity), teaching new methods of task performance (e.g., work-simplification procedures, specialized compensatory techniques), and provision of adaptive equipment (e.g., specialized or custom adaptive equipment; altering the shape, size, and/or weight of

task objects). In the context of using the adaptive occupation, adaptations and gradations are designed as "***longer term solutions***" ***to enable the client to compensate for ineffective actions***.

2. ***Propose solutions (offer alternative options)***: The proposed solutions are based on the principles and methods of adaptation discussed above. The occupational therapist, the client, and other members of the extended consultative partnership work together to creatively and collaboratively identify alternative or compensatory strategies or adaptations that are appropriate to the needs of the client. Proposing solutions and then evaluating them to ensure that they will be effective might best be viewed as "***the art and science of guided trial and error***."

3. ***Confirm that the adaptation will improve task performance***: As I pointed out above, proposing solutions and verifying that they will meet the needs of the client is a process often characterized by trial and error. The occupational therapist must ensure that the adaptation is reliable and safe and, through collaborative consultative partnerships, verify that the proposed adaptation is acceptable to the client and to others who will be impacted by the adaptation. Moreover, it is important that the occupational therapist determine that the adaptation will result in a task performance that is satisfying to the client and/or requires less effort, is more efficient, is more safe, reduces the client's need for assistance, and/or is more socially appropriate.

Education

Principles of education may be applied to persons with disabilities, caregivers, teachers, service extenders (aides or assistants), or other professionals. Determination of who may be the recipient of the learning process is established using the principles of collaborative consultation discussed above. The following principles have been modified and expanded from those originally presented by Trombly (1995c):[16]

1. ***Determine what the learner knows***: Learning can be conceptualized as occurring in phases. In the first phase, we come to ***understand*** basic concepts. For the person who sought/was referred for occupational therapy services, this phase includes (a) developing an understanding of what person, task, environmental, or societal factors

[16] See also Flinn and Radomski (2008) for an excellent review of general learning principles as applied to persons with physical disabilities. While their focus is on motor learning among persons with physical disabilities, I believe that they apply equally well to occupational performance.

facilitate and support or hinder and limit occupational performance; and (b) learning which strategies that may be more or less effective when implementing a task performance. In the second phase, the person builds on these basic concepts and uses them to analyze his or her own performance, and to implement trial and error attempts to improve task performance through adaptation or compensation. This phase can be viewed as one of ***problem-solving***. In the third phase, the person's application of understanding and problem-solving becomes ***automatic***; the person's ability to adapt or compensate ***becomes habitual and can be generalized to new situations and contexts***. Important components of the teaching-learning process, therefore, are education, practice, and generalization. When we initiate the principles of education as we apply the compensatory model, we begin by determining where on a continuum of learning the recipient of the education lies, and whether or not he or she has begun to use problem-solving strategies to overcome problems in performance.

2. ***Establish the learning objective***: The learning objective is not to be confused with the client's goals. That is, the learning objective is related to the expected outcomes of the educational methods that the occupational therapist is going to use to achieve the client's goals. Consider the following examples:

    - **Client goal #1**: Lars will brush his teeth with only occasional cueing and minimal inefficiency (e.g., organizing task objects, and without short pauses).
      Learning objective #1: Lars' partner will learn to effectively cue Lars.

    - **Client goal #2**: Edward will safely prepare a bowl of cold cereal and a glass of juice with minimal physical assistance.
      Learning objective #2: Edward's wife will learn to efficiently assist Edward.

    - **Client goal #3**: Joan will independently self-propel her wheelchair around her kitchen, experiencing only minimal increase in physical effort.
      Learning objective #3: Joan will learn to (a) lock and unlock her brakes at the appropriate time; and (b) position herself appropriately in relation to cupboards, counters, and the refrigerator door.

3. ***Choose teaching techniques congruent with what is to be taught***: When we use educational principles to teach our clients how to use adapted equipment or assistive

technology, or new alternative or compensatory strategies, and to become independent problem-solvers, it is important that we use methods that (a) are relevant to the client's current level of performance and learning, (b) are relevant to the client-centered performance context, (c) offer the just-right challenge, and (d) provide the needed structure to promote learning. These same principles are applied to caregivers and service extenders who need to learn how to assist a person with a disability.

4. ***Adapt the presentation to the learner's capabilities***: As we proceed to implement teaching strategies, we must adapt them according to the person's ability to learn. Persons with cognitive disabilities may be able to learn only specific tasks. Other people will learn to be independent problem-solvers capable of automatic generalization of the principles of adaptation that they have learned. Strategies such as breaking complex tasks down into parts, providing structure, or using clear and concrete verbal and nonverbal cues are among those we might consider. Whenever possible, our goal is to progress the learner from the understanding phase of learning, through problem-solving, to that of automatic generalization.

5. ***Train in safe use of the adaptation***: Once we determine appropriate teaching strategies to use, the recipient of the education is taught to use adapted equipment, how to perform a task using alternative strategies, or how to assist the client to perform a task by providing social or physical modifications to the task environment.

6. ***Provide opportunities for practice, considering context and schedule***: As we provide opportunities for the client to practice new alternative or compensatory strategies, it is important that we promote naturalistic contexts in which the client can try new solutions (either those we may suggest or those the client discovers through his or her own trial and error or problem-solving) and practice old solutions. Similar principles are applied when the learner is the caregiver or service extender, and he or she is provided opportunities to practice assisting a person with a disability. In all cases, it is imperative that the practice involves doing — active participation on the part of the client.

7. ***Offer useful feedback at the right time***: While our provision of feedback may include motivational feedback in the form of ***encouragement*** ("Go ahead, try

again"), ***general feedback*** ("Good, nice job"), and ***knowledge of results*** ("You spread the butter on the bread"), Trombly (1995c) suggested that specific feedback regarding the performance (i.e., ***knowledge of performance***), provided immediately after the completion of a task, may be more useful. Providing specific feedback regarding what was and was not correct about a performance ("You tipped the jar too far; the juice spilled") can help a person with a disability or the caregiver/service extender progress to the problem-solving and automatic stages of learning. Moreover, ***summary feedback*** provided after several trials may be more effective that immediate feedback provided after each trial (Flinn & Radomski, 2008).

8. ***Test (reevaluate) the learner in the appropriate context to confirm that learning has occurred***: Just as the learning objective differs from the client's goal, reevaluation to ensure that learning has occurred should not be likened to reevaluation of the client to ensure that enhanced occupational performance has occurred. Rather, this step involves verification that the learner demonstrates behavior indicating that he or she is able to safely and effectively implement the adaptation. Achievement of the learning objective may or may not result in the client's goal being achieved.

3.2.3 Principles of Acquisitional and Restorative Occupation

Direct or Indirect Intervention

Direct or indirect intervention is always accomplished through the application of the principles of selected acquisitional and restorative models (e.g., developmental, sensory integration, behavioral, biomechanical, Model of Human Occupation, neurodevelopmental) in the context of acquisitional and restorative occupation. Direct intervention is that which is provided by the occupational therapist. Indirect intervention is that which is provided by a parent, teacher, caregiver, or service extender after being trained to do so by the occupational therapist.

Consultation and Education

As with adaptive occupation, consultation in the context of acquisitional and restorative occupation is based on a collaborative relationship among equals. In the case of acquisitional and restorative occupation, however, the focus is on collaborating with the client to (a) identify appropriate occupations to focus on during intervention, and/or (b) determine the client's desired outcomes (i.e., goals) and what forms of intervention will be provided. The occupational therapist brings to the relationship his or her expertise as to the realistic foci of intervention and the client brings expertise related to his or her desired outcomes. Such ***collaboration may include the need to negotiate, especially when the client's desired outcomes are unrealistic or unethical, or when the person who sought/was referred for occupational therapy services and his or her caregiver or family have conflicting goals***. In such cases, the perspectives of neither the person nor others in the client constellation are ignored. Rather, it is acknowledged as the occupational therapist seeks to negotiate a more realistic solution with all members of the client constellation. Collaboration and negotiation among all members of the client constellation or client group can be critical for successful outcomes.

Education, as it pertains to acquisitional and restorative models, generally involves teaching a client to perform specific skills and then allowing the client to practice and generalize those skills in the contexts of different environments and different tasks. The principles of education discussed above are also applied here, but without specific application to compensation through adaptation. The main difference, therefore, is that in acquisitional and restorative occupation, practice is given more emphasis and/or is extended over longer periods of time.

Grade Occupations via Modification or Adaption of the Task Challenge

Grading (i.e., modifying or adapting) occupations is based on the principles of activity analysis and synthesis (Mosey, 1986). Unlike when the principles of adaptation are applied in the context of adaptive occupation, ***when principles of adaptation are applied in the context of acquisitional and restorative occupation, they are always applied to alter the challenge of the task so as to provide the just right-challenge and then to gradually increase that challenge as the client's person factors, body functions, and/or occupational skills improve***. Gradations of task complexity, size and weight of objects, intensity, duration, and resistance are among the methods used to improve person factors and body functions and/or occupational skills. Such gradations may be designed to progress along developmental (e.g., motor, social, cognitive) continua, or they may be based on principles derived from the acquisitional and restorative model being applied (e.g., gradations of resistance when applying biomechanical principles).

3.2.4 Principles of Occupation-based Education Programs

As noted above, education is a critical component of adaptive, acquisitional, and restorative occupation. Such education, provided as part of the client learning about how to use new adaptive or compensatory strategies (as part of adaptive occupation), or when engaged in learning and practicing occupational skills (as part of acquisitional occupation) or motor control, etc. (as part of restorative occupation), is not to be confused with education provided in the context of occupation-based education programs. As noted earlier, ***occupation-based education programs are always implemented in a lecture, seminar, or workshop format*** (see Figure 10). The principles of education, when applied to occupational-based education programs, are very similar to first four steps presented earlier, but are modified here to conform to the classroom-like settings were occupational-based programs are implemented.

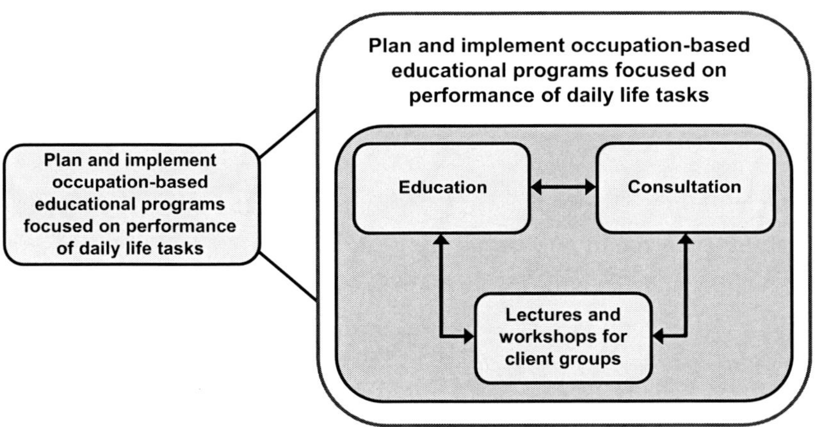

Figure 10. **Schematic representation of occupation-based educational programs.**

1. ***Determine what the learners know***: The first phase of learning involves the clients in the educational program developing an understanding of what person, task, environmental, or societal factors facilitate and support or hinder and limit their occupational performances, as well as learning what strategies the clients are using that may be more or less effective when performing daily life tasks. In the second

phase, the persons or others in the client constellations build on these basic concepts and use them to analyze their own performances, and to become aware of potential strategies they might use to achieve enhanced occupational performances and satisfaction with their occupational performances. ***When we initiate the principles of education within occupation-based education programs, we often begin with group discussions that enable us to determine where on a continuum of learning the recipients of the education lie, and whether or not they have begun to use problem-solving strategies to overcome problems in performance.***

2. ***Establish the learning objective***: In the case of occupation-based education programs, the learning objectives apply to the group as a whole, and are determined based on what the learners already know. As discussed earlier, it is critical not to confuse the learning objective with the clients' goals. It is also critical to keep in mind that the learning ***objective must be focused on occupation, not, for example, the understanding of one's illness***. The latter can be addressed in educational programs, but are not the responsibility or focus of the occupational therapist. That is, in many settings, occupational therapists participate in educational programs along with other team members. In such instances, a physician may address the nature of the illness, disease, or disability; the physical therapist may address issues related to physical activity and movement; and ***the occupational therapist addresses issues related to occupational performance (i.e., occupation-based education). In the absence of participation of the other members of the team, we must never be tempted to fulfill their role***. That is, we must maintain our focus on occupation.

3. ***Choose teaching techniques congruent with what is to be taught***: When we use educational principles within the context of occupation-based education programs, it is important that we use methods that (a) are relevant to the clients' current levels of performance and learning, (b) are relevant to their client-centered performance contexts, (c) offer the just-right challenge, and (d) provide the needed structure to promote learning. We must keep in mind, however, that in occupation-based education programs, the clients will have an opportunity to discuss strategies that they might try to implement later, but that ***specific training and practice in the use of adaptive equipment or compensatory strategies, occupational skills training, and training in relation to person factors or body functions are not part of occupation-based education programs***. That form of education is provided in the context of adaptive, acquisitional, or restorative occupation, respectively.

4. ***Adapt the presentation to the learner's capabilities***: As we proceed to implement occupation-based education programs, we must adapt them according to the clients' abilities to learn. Whenever possible, our goal is to progress the learners from the understanding phase of learning, through to problem-solving, and even automatic generalization.

4. OTIPM AS A REASONING MODEL FOR IMPLEMENTING COMPREHENSIVE OCCUPATIONAL THERAPY SERVICES — CASE EXAMPLE: BEV

A common concern expressed by occupational therapists has been related to our need for a conceptual model of practice that would enable us to better integrate theory, assessment, and intervention methods into our practices and to communicate with our colleagues about what it is that is unique about occupational therapy. In this chapter, I will present the OTIPM in more detail (see Chapter 1, Figure 5). This model not only helps us to better integrate theory, assessment, and intervention methods into occupational therapy practice, it also enables us to make the philosophical foundations of our profession a reality of everyday practice. That is, the OTIPM (a) unites practice and theory in an occupational framework, (b) stresses our use of a ***true top–down approach*** to assessment, and (c) provides us with a framework to guide our professional reasoning that leads to the implementation of ***occupation-based interventions*** for purposes of compensation, occupational skills training, restoration or development of person factors and body functions, and/or occupation-based education programs. In this process, the OTIPM provides a framework for making decisions about what evaluation methods to use, what occupational therapy or related models of practice to use, and when to use them in the evaluation and intervention planning process.

This point is worth clarifying further. In the course of our occupational therapy education, we are exposed to knowledge derived from a broad variety of sources. In our pre-occupational therapy courses, we learn concepts related to such diverse areas as human development, psychology, and neuroanatomy. In our occupational therapy education, we learn about specific approaches, frames of reference, and theories (collectively, models of practice), many of which were developed outside our profession. We also learn a broad range of knowledge and skills associated with the evaluation and intervention methods we use in practice. More often than not, such learning is broken up into discrete units and spread out across numerous courses. The same is often true when we take post-professional continuing or advanced education courses. As a result, rather than being integrated into a cohesive whole, learning becomes fragmented. ***A primary purpose for developing the OTIPM was to provide***

the learner with a structure for integrating such diverse knowledge and skills into the occupational therapy intervention process.

If we are to unite practice and theory in an occupational framework, we must conceptualize and implement practice in a manner that explicitly ties our professional reasoning and behavior to our unique focus on occupation as a therapeutic tool. I believe that the OTIPM provides us with a structure for realizing this objective.

In this chapter, I will use a ***case application of a woman named Bev***[17] to demonstrate how the OTIPM can be applied in practice. This case application is based on a collaborative experience I had with three occupational therapy graduate students as part of a Level I Fieldwork Placement. I will summarize our collaborative experience as we used the OTIPM to guide our professional reasoning to implement the evaluation, planning, and intervention phases of Bev's occupational therapy.

In addition to providing a structure for professional reasoning, the OTIPM provides us with a ***structure for systematic documentation that can support evidence-based practice and program evaluation***. Therefore, as part of my presentation of the case example (Bev), I will include our step-by-step process for documenting occupational therapy services. A detailed structure for comprehensive documentation is included in the Appendix, Section 8.2. The documentation included in this chapter will follow that structure.

4.1 Establish the Client-centered Performance Context

The first step of the OTIPM is to ***establish the client-centered performance context*** (see Chapter 1, Figure 5) The client-centered performance context provides the framework for understanding who is the client[18], what needs the client has, what the client does, and what problems the client has with performance of daily life tasks, including work, school, play, leisure, self-care (personal activities of daily living, PADL), and complex or instrumental activities of daily living (IADL; e.g., home maintenance, shopping, meal preparation). The goal, therefore, is to ***gather as much***

[17] The case example of Bev is adapted, with permission, from Fisher (2006a).

[18] As I noted in Chapter 1, in OTIPM, the term *client* is used to refer to a person, a client constellation, or a client group. In this chapter, Bev is the client. In another context, the client might be a student and his or her teacher or the educational team who has expressed concerns about the student's poor schoolwork performance; or it might be a woman with dementia, and her daughter and husband who are now the woman's caregivers. In yet another context, the client may be a company (administrators and employees, i.e., a client group) who are concerned about the prevention of work-related injuries.

information as is possible, in a relatively short period of time, related to the client's global client-centered performance context so as to obtain a general picture of the client's internal personal characteristics and the external factors that, together, comprise the context for the client's performance of daily life tasks. Once the client-centered performance context is established, the occupational therapist should have a good understanding of (a) the reason for the client's referral to occupational therapy, (b) the resources and limitations within the client-centered performance context, (c) the client's self-reported level of performance of daily life tasks, and (d) which tasks the client prioritizes as the initial targets for evaluation and potential intervention. I will discuss each of these outcomes of establishing the client-centered performance context in more detail, later, when I present the subsequent steps of the OTIPM.

4.1.1 Defining the Performance Context

As we consider the term *performance context*, we must keep in mind the premise that occupational performance unfolds as a transaction between a person and the environment as he or she enacts a task (see Figure 11). Therefore, if we are to establish the client-centered performance context, we must consider more than just the features of the task and the physical and social environments (cf. Christiansen & Baum, 1997; Dunn, Brown, & McGuigan, 1994; Haugen & Mathiowetz, 1995). We must also acknowledge that the person's motivational characteristics, roles, and underlying person factors and body functions are just as critical as are the task and the environment for establishing the context needed to understand why, and how, a person, a client constellation, or a group performs the tasks they do, and why certain aspects of the task performance may result in their experiencing difficulty or dissatisfaction.

More specifically, the performance context is comprised of both internal and external factors. ***Internal factors*** are those within the client, and ***external factors*** are those that are outside or external to the client (see Table 2). In total, the performance context is comprised of 10 dimensions. Some of them have components which are both internal and external to the client (i.e., role, cultural, and temporal dimensions). Each of these dimensions can have features that are resources which support the client's occupational performance, as well as features which limit the client's occupational performance. The content or focus of each dimension of the performance context is summarized in Table 3, in the form of ***key questions the occupational therapist must seek to answer***, not questions the occupational therapist is to ask.

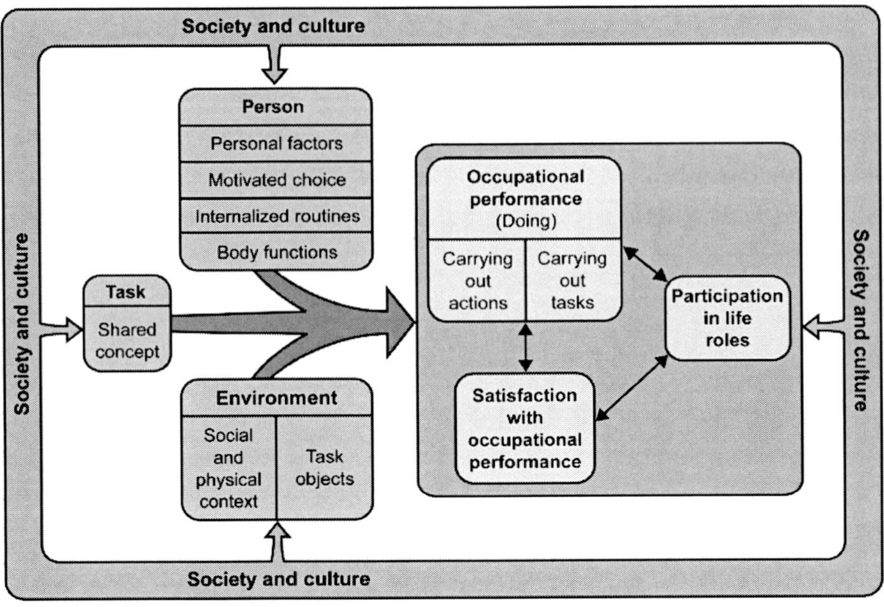

Figure 11. **Schematic representation of occupational performance unfolding as a transaction between the person and the environment as he or she enacts a task.**

Table 2 External and Internal Factors that Comprise the Client-centered Performance Context

External factors	Internal factors
Environmental	Role
Role	Cultural
Task	Motivational
Cultural	Body function
Social	Temporal (e.g., age)
Societal	Adaptive
Temporal (e.g., time of day, season)	

Table 3 Key Questions that Clarify the Content or Focus of the 10 Dimensions of the Client-centered Performance Context

Environmental dimension:

- When the client performs tasks,
  - Who is present?
  - What objects are used?
  - In what physical spaces does the client perform tasks?

Role dimension:

- What roles are important to the client?
- Are role-related tasks performed in a logical, timely, and socially appropriate manner?
- Are there any inconsistencies between the client's desired role behavior and
  - The client's actual engagement in role behavior?
  - The role behavior that is expected by society or desired by the client?

Motivational dimension:

- Do the client's values, interests, and goals provide meaning and a source of motivation for occupation?
- What are the client's priorities, hopes, and concerns for future occupational performance?
- Is there evidence that the client has a source of inner drive (e.g., spirituality, connections to others, a will to live)?

Task dimension:

- What tasks does the client report are ones the client needs and wants (or is expected by society) to perform?
- What are the characteristics of those tasks (e.g., complexity, duration, key elements)?

Cultural dimension:

- Are there shared cultural beliefs, values, and customs that influence:
  - Where the client performs tasks?
  - What tasks the client performs?
  - How the client performs tasks?
  - What tools and materials the client uses during task performance?

Social dimension:

- Does the client have connections and relationships with others?
- What is the extent and quality of collaboration that occurs between the client and others?

Societal dimension:

- What resources and restrictions must be considered?
  - Available services?
  - Economic factors, including needed funding for services?
  - Rules, regulations, and health care policies?
  - Societal attitudes?
  - Medical precautions?

Body function dimension:

- What information is included in the client's record related to the client's underlying physical, cognitive, and psychosocial capacities and impairments?
- During your informal observations of the client during the initial interview, what initial impressions did you have of the client's underlying physical, cognitive, and psychosocial capacities and impairments?
- What does this information tell you about the client's potential for recovery of underlying physical, cognitive, and psychosocial capacities and impairments?

Temporal dimension:

- What are the client's daily life routines?
- What is the client's current life stage?
- When relevant, have you considered the past, present, and future of all other dimensions?

Adaptation dimension:

- Is there any evidence that the client
  - Has modified behavior and/or adapted environments to overcome problems?
  - Is flexible and open to the idea of change?

4.1.2 Interrelatedness of the 10 Dimensions of the Client-centered Performance Context

The 10 dimensions of the client-centered performance context listed in Tables 2 and 3 are highly interrelated. As a result, the questions in Table 3 serve more as a guide to what information to seek (and not to seek) than as a specific structure for gathering information about the client. For example, consider a student who receives assistance within a regular classroom from an assistant. More specifically, she helps him with such schoolwork tasks such as writing and coloring, and with all of his ADLs (e.g., toileting, putting on and taking off his jacket before and after recess).

Just by obtaining this small piece of information about the student, we have ***simultaneously learned a little about four different dimensions*** because they are interrelated. First, we learned a bit about the ***environmental dimension*** (the assistant is a person who is present in the classroom during the student's school task performances), and we learned that the physical setting is a regular classroom, not, for example, a special education classroom. At the same time, we learned a little about the ***task and role dimensions*** (writing, coloring, toileting, and dressing are tasks the student needs to perform as part of his student role). Finally, we learned a bit about the ***societal dimension*** as the assistant is a resource provided by the school to students in need of supportive services.

4.1.3 Using the 10 Dimensions to Ensure that We Gather Comprehensive Information, Not as an Interview Guide

Because of this interrelatedness of the 10 dimensions of the client-centered performance context, it is important to keep in mind that ***we never ask the client a series of questions, moving systematically from one dimension to another***. That is, the 10 dimensions are ***not*** intended to be a structured guide to the interview, nor are they the direct basis for the questions we ask. ***Rather, we use the dimensions more as a framework to be sure we gather the information we need to learn about the client, determine the client's goals and priorities, and plan and implement client-centered intervention***.

It is also important to point out that another reason we would not want to use the questions in Table 3 as an interview guide is that the questions may have little or no meaning to our clients, or they may be too threatening. For example, it would generally be inappropriate to say to a client, "Tell me about your culture — does your culture influence what tasks you perform and how you do them?" or "Can you tell me a little more about your spirituality?" Such questions are too broad and too vague. Rather, at this point in the professional reasoning process, the cultural dimension is more related to the importance of our ***being aware of, listening for, and accepting cultural differences among our clients***. We also need to know enough about the cultural expectations for performance to be able to make sound judgments related to whether or not the client performs tasks in a logical manner.

The primary value of using the 10 dimensions is that they provide us with a ***structure for summarizing all of the background information that we gather*** and ensure that we have gathered all information needed both to understand the client's current situation and concerns, and later, to clarify or interpret why the client may be experiencing difficulty with certain occupational performances. Moreover, we must remain acutely aware that additional information will always need to be gathered as we establish the ***specific*** client-centered performance context for each daily life task that becomes a focus for further evaluation and/or intervention.

4.1.4 Defining the Global versus Specific Client-centered Performance Context

The client-centered performance pertains to the context within which the person and others in the client constellation actually perform those tasks they perform. When we first meet the client, our goal is to begin to conceptualize the client-centered performance context at a broad, ***global*** level. That is, our initial focus in more on gathering the information needed to build a broad picture of what tasks the client needs and wants to perform, what tasks the client does perform, where the client performs them, why the client performs them, and how the client performs them. Ultimately, however, our focus will be on the ***specific*** client-centered performance context — the specific context within which the client enacts each work, school, play, leisure, self-care, or IADL task the client performs and prioritizes for further evaluation. As a result, the context for a person's bathing will differ somewhat from that for dressing or meal preparation. Moreover, the context for bathing will vary over time depending on whether or not the person chooses to wash his hair, how he is feeling, and so on. Each day, we get up and get dressed, but the context is never exactly the same — ***the internal and external factors within our own client-centered performance contexts vary from day to day, moment to moment***.

4.1.5 Linking to Other Models of Practice

As the occupational therapist establishes the client-centered performance context, he or she may choose to link to other conceptual models of practice. In doing so, the occupational therapist should ***not*** have the specific intention of using the same model(s) to guide this phase of the evaluation process as he or she might decide to use later as a guide to intervention. While the occupational therapist may later choose to use the same model(s) to guide both the evaluation and intervention phases, the decision as to what model(s) to choose for intervention is always deferred until after the occupational therapist has defined/clarified or interpreted the cause of the client's ineffective goal-directed actions of task performance.

The advantage of linking to other models of practice when establishing the client-centered performance context is for the professional reasoning process (and ultimately, the client) to benefit from existing theory when elaborate models have already been developed that more specifically explain one or more dimensions of the client-centered performance context. For example, in Bev's case, we could have chosen to link to the Model of Human Occupation (Kielhofner, 2008). For example, Kielhofner's conceptualization of the physical and social environment in terms of demands and constraints versus opportunities and resources, and how each help to form occupational performance, provides the occupational therapist with theoretical principles that extend beyond that of the OTIPM. In a similar manner, we could have chosen to use Kielhofner's conceptualization of the volition subsystem if we had felt that it would have enriched our understanding of Bev's sources of motivation for occupational performance. We would need to keep in mind, however, that Kielhofner does not consider spirituality as a source of motivation.

The purpose of linking is to draw upon existing theory (rather than replicate it here) when other compatible models already exist. Both the OTIPM and the Model of Human Occupation (Kielhofner, 2008)

> *are practice theories in their own right. . . . Each maintains its integrity by retaining its identity as a distinct theory. Rather, what we are proposing is that the practice of occupational therapy can be enhanced by linking compatible theories when the needs of the client extend beyond the specific domain addressed by the primary theory that guides practice.* (Kielhofner & Fisher, 1991, p. 31)

4.1.6 Establishing the Client-centered Performance Context — Initial Referral

Establishing the client-centered performance context typically begins with an initial referral and/or telephone contact with a client who is seeking occupational therapy services. The initial referral or initial telephone contact serves as the starting point of the occupational therapy intervention process. The referral commonly includes some background information about the person or group that is referred to occupational therapy (e.g., age, diagnoses), as well as information about why the client was referred (e.g., the client's problem, what type of evaluation and/or intervention is being requested). Similarly, when clients seek our services, they commonly provide some information about themselves and why they seek our services.

While the initial referral may include a reason for the referral, ***the stated reason is not always clearly related to our unique role and our focus on occupation*** — the ability of the client to perform those tasks the client needs and wants to perform, and to be able to perform them with satisfaction. For example, a person might be referred for gait training or muscle strengthening. In other instances, the referral may request occupational therapy services that are not relevant to the client's needs or problems. In such cases, we must keep in mind that ***we have an ethical responsibility to retain the focus of our evaluations and interventions on occupation***, those task performances that the client needs and wants to perform, and inform the client about our unique professional role and what services we can ethically offer (AOTA, 2005; FSA, 2005).

4.1.7 Establishing the Client-centered Performance Context — Initial Occupational Therapy Interview

Once we receive a referral and/or have had initial telephone contact with a client seeking occupational therapy services, the next step is to meet the client.[19] Through an initial occupational therapy interview (and informal observations during the interview), we continue to construct an initial, ***global picture*** of the client-centered performance context. Ultimately, however, it is the interview that becomes the key source of information that enables us to understand the person and others in the client constellation, and their needs and concerns, from their own perspectives — the insider's point of view.

When a person lacks the ability to communicate and/or is unable to express clearly his or her needs and problems, the occupational therapist must talk with others who have needed information related to the client-centered performance context. Such persons may include family members or other professionals (e.g., social workers) who are ***not*** part of the client constellation. Whether the other persons whom we interview to find out about the person who seeks/is referred to occupational therapy are within or outside the client constellation does not matter, ***we must take very precaution to learn about the person who seeks/is referred, and how his or her concerns and priorities may differ from those who are reporting on his or her behalf***. Obviously, we also

[19] If the occupational therapist has available the client's record, the therapist would usually implement a chart review before seeing the client.

want to learn about the concerns and priorities of all of the persons who are members of the client constellation.

Learning more about the client, the tasks that are most important to the client, the meaning of those tasks, and the nature of the contexts within which those task performances are likely to be enacted requires taking the time and effort to establish the client-centered performance context. This step is critical, and it must occur, even under the pressures of cost containment, reduced duration of care, staff cuts, and increased accountability. ***Taking the time needed to establish the client-centered performance context will result in overall outcomes being enhanced and overall costs reduced*** (Bowen, 1996; Neistadt, 1995). Our use of active listening skills will also result in greater therapeutic rapport, better understanding of the client, and, in turn, enhanced motivation and greater compliance (Kerr, 1999).

Ideally, the interview progresses naturally, with the occupational therapist and the client engaging in a conversation. It is often preferable to have no predetermined plan or order for the interview, and instead, follow the lead of the client. Using structured interviews such as the *Canadian Occupational Performance Measure* (COPM) (Law et al., 2005) or the *ADL Taxonomy* (Törnqvist & Sonn, 2001) later in the interview can, however, help the client identify which task performances are of most concern and which ones the client wants to prioritize for evaluation. This step will be discussed below.

While it is important to follow the lead of the client, it is also important to keep the interview focused on the information needed, and to avoid delving into topics that are irrelevant — doing so is contrary to time- and cost-effective occupational therapy services. It is, therefore, desirable to bring to the interview a set of key, open-ended questions (often presented in the form of open-ended statements) that the occupational therapist can use help guide the interview, while allowing for it to progress naturally, and in a flexible manner. Some ***examples*** of some key "questions" are the following:

1. Do you know about occupational therapy; have you ever worked with another occupational therapist?
2. Can you describe for me a typical day?
3. Can you tell me more about your morning routine?
4. What challenges are you experiencing with the different activities you engage in?
5. What is it about that activity that makes it challenging?
6. Is there anything you'd like to do that you are not doing now?

7. Are there people available that can help you if you need it? Your family? Neighbors?
8. What activities would you like to work on now in occupational therapy?

Again, these are just examples. Obviously, they would need to be modified and/or expanded so as to address different settings, client concerns, and so on. For example, if the client is a student and a teacher, the occupational therapist might ask the teacher to describe her classroom rather than a typical day. Or, if a client is referred for a work evaluation, the occupational therapist might choose to begin by saying, "I understand that you have some concerns about work. Can you tell me about them?"

In general, our initial questions should be designed to be broad and not overly specific. In most instances, we can anticipated that the client's answers to our initial guiding questions will lead to more specific questions we will want to ask the client so that we would gain a clear picture of the client's performance context.

A final point that is important to keep in mind, when implementing initial occupational therapy interviews, is finding a balance between not gathering enough information and going into too much detail, too early in the occupational therapy intervention process. It is often the case that some of the information we gather is not relevant. We must keep in mind, therefore, that ***cost-effective interviewing and information-gathering requires that we recognize early (a) when it would not be appropriate to take the time to gather more information or delve into detail about some topic that the client might raise, (b) when it would be more appropriate to defer exploring a topic in more detail, and (c) when to redirect the client so as to keep the client focused on sharing the relevant and helpful information we need to understand the client's performance context***. The *initial* occupational therapy interview rarely takes more 20 to 30 minutes to complete, provided the occupational therapist follows these guidelines.

4.2 Case Example: Bev — Establishing the Client-centered Performance Context

4.2.1 Bev: Initial Referral

Bev was referred to us by her daughter because of concerns that Bev was experiencing difficulty at home getting around her apartment safely and managing simple meal preparation tasks. In requesting our services, Bev's daughter told me the following information, which I shared with the students. Bev had recently moved into an independent living complex following hospitalization and a subsequent period in a nursing home. Apparently, Bev had been hospitalized on several occasions over the past several years, but I was not sure of the reason for her most recent hospitalization. I learned from her daughter that Bev had received occupational therapy services from a home health occupational therapist after returning to her apartment, but that occupational therapy was discontinued after only a few visits.

4.2.2 Bev: Preparing for the Occupational Therapy Interview

With these thoughts in mind, we began to prepare for our initial visit and our occupational therapy interview. We knew that we wanted to gather as much relevant information a possible in the shortest possible time. We started, therefore, by considering the 10 dimensions of the client-centered performance context, and developed a few key guiding questions we hoped to have Bev answer. When we met with Bev, we knew we would need to reword them, sometimes simplify them, before asking them of Bev. For example, after introducing ourselves and telling her that we were occupational therapists (one occupational therapist and three occupational therapy students), we originally planned to say to Bev, "Your daughter mentioned that you might be experiencing some challenges preparing meals. Can you tell us more about that?" Based on her reply, we would need to be prepared to probe deeper so as to gather progressively more specific information. Or, if it felt more appropriate, we knew we could transition by asking her, "Did you work on meal preparation with any of your prior occupational therapists?" If she responded affirmatively, we could probe deeper by asking, "What did you work on that you found to be helpful?" We also realized that we could easily transition from talking about meal preparation to asking Bev, "Are you able to manage your toileting, bathing, and dressing by yourself, or does someone help you with any of these tasks?" We could also probe deeper by asking, "Is there anything about these tasks that you are concerned about?" The point here is that we wanted to progress the interview as if it were a naturalistic conversation, one that would (a) be comfortable and nonthreatening for Bev; (b) ensure a good understanding of Bev, her circumstances, her concerns, and her priorities; and (c) would yield for us the information we needed to be able to best help her.

While we did not want to specifically ask Bev about each dimension (e.g., "Can you tell me about your roles?"), we did review them so that we would remember the scope of the information we would want to gather. We also made special note of the temporal dimension to remind us to consider the past, present, and future as we gathered information about all of the other dimensions (e.g., her roles, where she lives, what services she receives).

Finally, we reasoned that, consistent with a true top–down approach to assessment, we did not plan to formally assess any of Bev's person factors or body functions. For example, we our plan was to avoid asking her any questions aimed at assessing her cognitive functions, nor did we plan to ask her to reach, bend, or move her body in order to screen for limitations in strength, range of motion, or endurance. Rather, at this stage, we wanted to know only enough about Bev's diagnoses and/or medical history to learn if there were any medical precautions we needed to be aware of — we did not have access to her medical record, otherwise, we would have gathered that information from her record and not planned to ask Bev for this information. Otherwise, our plan was to rely solely on our informal observations as we carried out our initial interview.

4.2.3 Bev: Initiating the Home Visit and Implementing the Occupational Therapy Interview

I called Bev after receiving her occupational therapy referral to make arrangements for a time for us to come see her. The telephone conversation and the opportunity to see where she lived provided us with a great deal of information about Bev's global client-centered performance context, even before we began to ask her our questions. Over the phone, she gave me clear and detailed directions about where her apartment building was located, where to park, and how to come into her building and find her apartment. When we arrived for our initial visit, she greeted us with a cheerful smile. We noticed that she was in a wheelchair and that she looked frail. She also had plastic tubing with a nasal cannula that provided her with supplemental oxygen.

As we entered her apartment, we walked past the bathroom and the bedroom and into the living room. The five of us, three students sitting in the only chairs, myself sitting on the floor, and Bev sitting in her wheelchair, barely fit into her small living room. In fact, Bev sat more in the adjoining kitchen than in the living room. Looking into her kitchen, we wondered if it was possible for her to maneuver her wheelchair to turn around in the limited space between the cabinets on either side.

As we walked past her bathroom, we observed that it appeared to be well equipped. There was a raised toilet seat and a safety frame around the toilet. In the shower/bathtub were grab bars, a hand-held shower head, and a bathtub transfer bench. Her small bedroom had a hospital-style electric bed and there was a commode beside the bed. Again, there appeared to be little room to maneuver a wheelchair between the bed and the closet or the door, and it was clear that it would not be possible to get around the far side of the bed in either a wheelchair or by using a walker.

We had no difficulty engaging Bev in conversation. In fact, our greater challenge was to keep her on topic. As she knew we were occupational therapists (and despite our initial plan), she began by telling us about her experiences with her many previous occupational therapists. "I've had some good ones and some that were not so good. The good ones put me through my paces, but there were some who did not do therapy."

Her most recent home health occupational therapist had authorization to see Bev for six visits. She had spent most of her first five visits talking with Bev about the news of the day or about church. She also gave Bev a small green foam ball to squeeze to exercise her fingers and to place under her feet to exercise her legs, and she tied Thera-Band® to Bev's wheelchair so that Bev could exercise her upper limbs. During her final visit, the occupational therapist advised Bev to put her laundry basket in the closet so that she would have more room to maneuver her wheelchair around in the bedroom. About her experience, Bev said, "Some visiting is a joy, but it is not therapy. Time could have been better spent and money used more wisely."

Bev also insisted on recounted for us her medical history. Slightly more than 3 years ago, Bev was admitted to the hospital with pneumonia. She was in an intensive care unit and on a ventilator. During that time, three blocked arteries in her legs resulted in decreased oxygen to her feet. They "turned black," and she had to have partial foot amputations of both feet. Once she stabilized medically, she was fitted with special shoes and taught to walk with a walker. She was discharged 3 months later. Six months after her discharge, Bev fell and broke her right hip while reaching for something, and was readmitted to the hospital. When discharged, she transitioned to a nursing home for rehabilitation and then she opted to move, temporarily, into an assisted living facility. Over the next 14 months she had several more hospitalizations because of congestive heart failure, pneumonia, and bronchitis.

Then, 6 months before our initial visit, just as she was preparing to move back into the independent living complex, she walked through an automatic door that closed on her. She fell and fractured her right distal femur. She was readmitted to the hospital, transitioned to a nursing home for rehabilitation, and then to her apartment in the independent living complex. A few days later, she began experiencing acute pain in her lower back. A week later she was back in the hospital and diagnosed with compression fractures of her lower lumbar spine. Once again, she was transitioned back to the nursing home. She returned to her apartment 2 months before our initial visit. Bev described these past few years as a "smorgasbord of bad health."

As the conversation proceeded, we probed further so as to gather the information we would need to establish the client-centered performance context. Again, we did not specifically ask Bev about each of the 10 dimensions of the client-centered performance context. Instead, we asked simple, clear questions that naturally proceeded from what we had just discussed, yet remained focused on gathering the information we needed, and avoided topics that were not directly related to the information we needed. That is, as much as possible, we tried to avoid having Bev discuss information or aspects of her life tangential to that necessary for purposes of planning and implementing client-centered occupational therapy. In a very short time (25 minutes), we learned a great deal of information that provided us with a framework for understanding, evaluating, and later interpreting her occupational performances.

We concluded our interview by administering the COPM, which took an additional 25 to 30 minutes. Administering the COPM, however, gave Bev the opportunity to more clearly identify her priorities for occupational therapy services.

Bev told us that she is satisfied overall with the tasks she performs and the assistance she receives. For example, she is generally satisfied with having a homemaker who comes once a week to clean her apartment, change the sheets on her bed, and do her laundry, but she wants to be able to do more of her cooking herself. Bev would like to be able to prepare warm meals, but she is concerned about safety in the kitchen. With regard to self-care, she is satisfied with receiving daily help from a home health aide who helps Bev with bathing, makes Bev's bed, and sometimes prepares Bev's breakfast. With regard to bathing, Bev expressed concerns about a fall risk when she is standing, but feels "safe and secure" when the home health aide is assisting her. Bev is able to toilet independently during the day, but because she cannot walk to the toilet without her shoes on, at night she uses the bedside commode. The home health aide empties Bev's commode each day. Bev's only expressed concern with self-care was related to being able to put on her right shoe and get her clothes from her closet — both tasks are currently physically effortful and "take too much time." When we asked her about getting out more, she told us that she feels that she currently is too weak to tolerate going out any more than she does. When she is stronger, she would like to participate more in the activities that are available in her building, return to church, and get out more for shopping and to restaurants. While her daughter takes her shopping and out to eat, Bev would like to get out more often.

Later, after we had returned to the university, the students and I used the key questions in Table 3 to organize all of the information we had gathered from Bev's daughter, our interview, and our informal observations of Bev and her apartment. Typically, my notes are comprised of a few short phrases under each dimension — the time constraints of most workplaces do not allow for more. In Bev's case, however, we included more detailed information so as to enhance the reader's understanding of both Bev and the 10 dimensions of her global performance context (see Table 4).

Table 4 Notes Written by the Occupational Therapy Students that Summarize the 10 Dimensions of Bev's Global Performance Context

Environmental dimension[20]

Lives in three room apartment (bedroom, living room, kitchen) in an independent living complex — well-equipped with durable adaptive equipment (e.g., bedside commode, grab bars in the bathroom); very limited space for maneuvering wheelchair or working in the kitchen; options for Bev's relocating to a larger apartment are not available.

Aide present to assist with bathing, makes Bev's bed, and sometimes prepare Bev's breakfast. Homemaker present to clean apartment, change sheets on bed, do laundry. Daughter present when she goes shopping or out to restaurants. Plays table games with grandchildren.

[20] As I noted in Section 4.2.3, these notes are much more detailed than might be needed or realistic in practice. For example, our actual notes for the Environmental dimension were as follows: "*3 room apt., indep living; small & crowded. Commode, grab bars, bath bench – bathroom. Assist from aide for bathing, making bed, preparing breakfast. Homemaker – cleans apt., changes sheets, does laundry. Daughter – assists with shopping, eating out. Grandchildren – cards, games.*"

Table 4 Continued

Role dimension

Bev is a self-maintainer, home-maintainer, mother, and grandmother. She has had past roles and hopes to regain as future roles as an active church-goer and social activity participant. Daughter reports Bev's self care tasks are performed in appropriate ways, given her level of disability, but cooking is unsafe. Bev reports some inconsistencies in self-maintainer role (desires being able to put on her right shoe and get her clothes from her closet more efficiently and with less effort), home-maintainer role (desires being able to do cooking independently and safely), and social activity participant role (feels she currently is too weak to tolerate going out, but when she is stronger, would like to participate more in activities available in her building, return to church, and get out more for shopping and to restaurants).

Motivational dimension

Interests include church, social activities, watching football, and playing table top and card games with her grandchildren. ADL and leisure seem to be the focus of Bev's current (and future) concerns. Attending church is a future concern. She wants to do more for herself, and she appeared to have realistic views of both her need for assistance and her potential to do more. Likens self to the Little Engine that Could *(Piper, 1930), stating that "If you've tried, you haven't failed." Her belief in God appears to provide a sense of hope; she expressed gratitude for God's gifts: "I asked God for all things so I could enjoy life. God gave me life so I could enjoy all things."*

Task dimension

Needs or desires to perform bathing, toileting, dressing, cooking, shopping, eating out, attending church, playing table top games and cards, socializing, watching football on television, and managing her oxygen tubing so that is does not "get tangled up in my wheelchair."

Cultural dimension

No apparent discrepancies between Bev's cultural beliefs, values, and customs and where and how she performs daily life tasks beyond the restrictions and modifications she has made as a result of her disabilities.

Social dimension

Satisfied with the assistance she is receiving from the home health aide and the homemaker; degree of collaboration unknown. Given that she is satisfied with the assistance she is receiving from the home health aide and the homemaker, we assumed her relationships with them are satisfactory. Daughter and grandchildren visit regularly; a friend who lives in the same building checks in on her every day; and she is visited by the home health aide, the homemaker, and the physical therapist. While her daughter takes her shopping and out to eat, Bev would like to get out more often. Finally, Bev has no social contact with her former husband.

Table 4 Continued

Bev's social contacts otherwise seemed to be limited. Seems to have had only occasional contact with her pastor, nor is she interested in his coming more often. While she used to be connected more to the other residents in her building through her active participation in social activities (e.g., monthly dinners, games), she stated that she was not physically able to participate now. Her hope that she might become involved again was indicated by her saying, "That too will come in due time."

Societal dimension

Bev is fairly well connected to available community resources: receives home delivery of one meal per day, home health aide comes every day for 1 hour each weekday and 1/2 hour on weekends, homemaker comes once each week. Uses bedside commode; the home health aide empties Bev's commode each day. Has had physical therapy two times a week since returning to her apartment, and anticipates physical therapist will continue to come for 1 more month. The main focus of her physical therapy has been increasing her endurance walking with her walker as she returns to full weight-bearing on her right leg.

Her pastor visits her once every 6 to 8 weeks. She is not receiving any help from members of her congregation, nor does she seem to feel the need for such connections. She would like to return to going to church, but stated, "That too will come in due time"; she indicated that she was not interested in getting a ride to church from anyone, including her daughter.

Relevant economic factors include the fact that she is on Medicaid as well as Medicare. Her current monthly income is very limited, and barely covers her expenses for medications, rent, utilities, home delivery of one meal per day, groceries, and household supplies. She has very little money left over after to pay for her much enjoyed social outings of shopping or eating out, much less for additional adaptive equipment or alterations to her apartment that might make task performances easier for her.

Implicit and explicit medical precautions are related to partial weight-bearing on her right leg, her limited endurance, and her need for supplemental oxygen.

Body function dimension

Significant history for congestive heart failure, pneumonia, and bronchitis. Currently uses oxygen (2 liters/day, 24 hours/day). Also has a significant history for fractures to her right hip and right distal femur, bilateral partial foot amputations, and lumbar compression fractures. Her memory and judgment appear to be intact. She appears to have no psychosocial problems and her current mood appears to be good. Bev is very frail and has limited endurance. We suspect that she has movement restrictions in her lower trunk and right hip and knee, and poor endurance that are affecting her performance of ADL tasks.

The chronic nature of her cardiopulmonary and musculoskeletal impairments suggest limited potential for full recovery, but we feel that she has potential to regain strength and endurance to a level close to that she had before her last injury and subsequent hospitalization.

Table 4 Continued

Temporal dimension
Bev is an older adult, 66 years of age. Her major work experience has been as a homemaker. She was married for 34 years, and was divorced 14 years ago. Finally, her transition into her older years occurred within the context of a significant medical history, including pneumonia, congestive heart failure, fracture of her right hip, and fractures to her lumbar spine.

Adaptation dimension
Appears to be a person who has flexible and open to change based on her comments (e.g., "If you've tried, you haven't failed"; and "I asked God for all things so I could enjoy life. God gave me life so I could enjoy all things"). Her realistic sense of self and her potential, along with her history of "persevering" despite multiple health problems, also suggests that she has adapted to changes in her life.

4.2.4 Bev: Who Is the Client?

As we interviewed Bev, we asked her about the people she has contact with and who helps her with her daily life task performances. Among them were her daughter, the homemaker, and the home health aide. I had talked with her daughter, and she had expressed no occupational performance concerns related to her mother. We reasoned, therefore, that Bev's daughter, while a significant source of information for us and a support for Bev, was not part of Bev's client constellation. Moreover, at least from Bev's perspective, the homemaker and the aide appeared to have no occupational performance concerns related to helping Bev. Therefore, we tentatively concluded that only Bev was our client. In so doing, our plan was to remain open to the idea that the aide, who was the person who was most involved in helping Bev, may actually be experiencing problems in relation to helping Bev. If we were to learn that this was the case, the aide would become part of Bev's client constellation.

4.3 Develop Therapeutic Rapport and Collaborative Relationships

When the occupational therapist meets the client and implements an occupational therapy interview to establish the client-centered performance context, he or she also begins the critical step of developing ***therapeutic rapport*** (Price, 2009; Tickle-Degnen, 2008). "Rapport is the process of establishing and maintaining a comfortable, unconstrained relationship of mutual confidence and respect between an occupational therapist and client" (Mosey, 1981, p. 96). Rapport has to do with the quality of the interaction between the occupational therapist and the client, and how this relationship affects the client's engagement in the intervention process (Tickle-Degnen). The development of a strong therapeutic relationship "requires that two people come to understand, trust, and respect one another and create shared meanings about what the therapy process means for the person's life and future" (Price, 2009, p. 329).

As the occupational therapist establishes the client-centered performance context and therapeutic rapport, he or she also begins the process of developing a ***collaborative (consultative) partnership*** between the client and the therapist that continues to develop throughout the entire time they work together (see the lighter grey arrows, Figure 5, Chapter 1). The occupational therapist brings to this partnership expertise related to available intervention strategies and knowledge related to potential outcomes. The client brings expertise related to his or her values, interests, goals, and priorities. If the collaborative partnership is to be effective, there must be open sharing of each other's motivations and rationales (Bowen, 1996). ***Letting go of our own personal goals for the client, while focusing on those of the client, can be a critical step in the process*** (Fisher, 1994; Tickle-Degnen, 2008). How we carry out the initial interview with the client to establish the client-centered performance context can also be critical. Probing too deeply, too quickly, especially into sensitive areas, can threaten the possibility of establishing the level of trust needed for open sharing. As Einhorn (2003, p. 81) said, "If I were to reformulate the golden rule. . . ." it would say, "you should attempt to meet [your clients] as they want to be met."

4.4 Case Example: Bev — Develop Therapeutic Rapport and a Collaborative Relationship

During our interview, Bev readily engaged in conversation, and openly shared with us her concerns and priorities. Early on in our conversation, it became clear to us that it was important for her to recount her extensive medical history. As part of developing trust and rapport, we felt that it was best to allow her to do so. Once she had done so, we remained constantly aware of the need to try to keep our conversation with Bev focused on occupation and relevant aspects of her performance context.

As we listened to her describe her past history and current problems with occupational performance, we expressed empathy and respect for Bev and what she had been through. As part of showing respect, we expressed no concerns about

Bev's desire to continue to receive help from others. Moreover, through simple gestures such as nodding and laughing at her jokes, we conveyed to Bev that we were actively listening to what she had to say. Reciprocally, as she seemed quite aware that much of her prior experiences with occupational therapists had been "less than ideal," and she looked forward to some "real occupational therapy," we sensed that she also was engaged in our discussion, and understood what we had to offer. Our overall sense was that Bev felt that she could openly express her concerns and desires, and that we would respond to her needs and desires, not our own. For example, at the end of our interview, we worked together to summarize the key areas of occupational performance that Bev had described as being problems, and we collaboratively decided how to proceed, given her priorities.

4.5 Identify the Resources and Limitations within the Client-centered Performance Context

After the occupational therapist has gathered information related to the 10 dimensions needed to establish the client-centered performance context (see Table 4), he or she is ready to summarize that information. That is, when the occupational therapist uses the OTIPM as a guide to professional reasoning, that information is summarized in two parts (a) resources and limitations within the client-centered performance context, and (b) identify and prioritize reported strengths and problems of occupational performance. The first component, ***resources and limitations within the client-centered performance context***, provides the occupational therapist with important background information that can be documented in the client's record and/or report of occupational therapy services.[21] The occupational therapist will also reflect back on this background information later in the occupational therapy intervention process when it is time to define/clarify or interpret the cause of the client's problems with occupational performance (see vertical dotted line in Figure 5, Chapter 1). At this phase of the intervention process, however, ***the occupational therapist focuses in on what aspects of the background information are important to document in the client's record***.

What the occupational therapist chooses to document may depend upon the structure of the client records in the setting where the occupational therapist works. For

[21] Most commonly, even if others in the client constellation are the primary focus on our interventions, documentation is placed in the record and/or evaluation report of the person who sought/was referred to occupational therapy.

example, if the occupational therapy record is separate from the documentation of other members of the team, the occupational therapist may want to include a bit more information than if all members of the team document in the same record. If, as is often the case, all members of the team document in the same record, there may be little or no need to repeat information that is already documented (e.g., age, diagnosis, living situation).[22]

4.6 Case Example: Bev — Identify the Resources and Limitations of the Client-centered Performance Context

After we read through our notes summarizing the information we had gathered related to the strengths and limitations of Bev's performance context (see Table 4), we began to document what we felt was the most important information we had gathered (see Documentation Example 1). As this was our initial evaluation, we wanted to provide a "picture of who is Bev" and why she was referred to us. When we documented Bev's background information and reason for referral, we wanted to limit our documentation to a few sentences, preferably, not more than five or six. We also wanted to maintain our focus on occupation-related background information that would provide support for the Bev's need for, and potential to benefit from, occupational therapy. For example, we were aware that if we indicated that Bev has good support from her daughter, we would provide a signal to any third party payees (e.g., private or national insurance) that she had good potential to benefit from any services we might provide. Moreover, since third party payees are often concerned about the provision of expensive services, we wanted to mention the services she currently is receiving, in the event that occupational therapy services might decrease somewhat her current level of need. Finally, beyond a short summary of her primary medical condition, we knew that it would not be appropriate to write anything about Bev's underlying body functions or limitations. That is, we reasoned that we wanted to document in an "occupation-first" manner, and not discuss Bev's underlying impairments until after we had documented more about her current status in relation to occupational performance.

---

[22] All documentation examples in this chapter were written in a format that assumes that they are independent occupational therapy reports, such as an occupational therapist might give to a client and/or to a third party payee.

4.7 Identify and Prioritize Reported Strengths and Problems of Occupational Performance

The second outcome of the information-gathering process implemented when the occupational therapist establishes the client-centered performance context is to ***summarize what task performances are strengths and which ones are problems, from the perspective of the client.*** Again, this information comes from the initial interview. When appropriate, the administration of the COPM (Law et al., 2005) or the ADL Taxonomy (Törnqvist & Sonn, 2001) serve as excellent tools that the occupational therapist can use to enable the client to self-identify what task performances the person or others in the client constellation perceive to be strengths or problems. That is, both tools are designed to provide a structure that can help the client identify and prioritize important problems with occupational performance.

Documentation Example 1: Bev: Initial Occupational Therapy Evaluation, Part I — Background Information and Reason for Referral

Background Information and Reason for Referral

Bev is a 66-year-old female currently living alone in a subsidized apartment following hospitalization. Enjoys games, watching football, social activities, and family. Services include daily home health aide, weekly homemaker, and home delivery of one meal per day. Home equipped with raised toilet seat, toilet safety frame, grab bars and extended bathtub transfer bench in bathtub, electric hospital bed, and bedside commode; supportive daughter provides community mobility. Past medical history significant for congestive heart failure, fractures to right hip and distal femur, and bilateral partial foot amputations. Referred due to "difficulty" and safety risk managing daily living tasks.

While both the COPM and ADL Taxonomy can help the client and occupational therapist to retain a focus on occupation, and not the client's underlying body functions or person factors, both also have limitations. The COPM is limited more by the interview skills and insight of the occupational therapist than by the tool itself. If, for example, the person mentions that one of her main concerns is lack of strength and coordination in her right hand, there is nothing to limit the occupational therapist from recording that information and later allowing the person to include diminished strength and coordination in her list of priorities. Strength and coordination, however, are not occupational performances. If the client reports problems with strength and coordination, the occupational therapist must follow-up and ask the client, "What tasks performances do you find challenging because of your limited strength and coordination?" Obviously, if the occupational therapist does not retain a focus on occupation and redirect the client, ***the risk becomes the loss of our ethical responsibility to retain the focus of our practice on occupation***.

When the occupational therapist uses the ADL Taxonomy, with its focus on self-care (PADL) and IADL, there is less risk of losing a focus on occupation. Rather, the risk becomes not expanding the interview (or optional self-report when the ADL Taxonomy is used) to other areas of occupation, including leisure, play, work, and school. Finally, both tools can only be used with persons who are able to actively engage in the interview process.

Returning to the step of *identifying and prioritizing reported strengths and problems with occupational performance*, task performances that support the client's role behavior are ***strengths of occupational performance***. Those that the client experiences as problematic, with which the person or others in the client constellation experience dissatisfaction, or that hinder their role behavior are ***problems of occupational performance***. Task performances are problematic when they require increased effort, are inefficient, are unsafe (or potentially unsafe), require verbal or physical assistance to be performed, and/or are socially inappropriate. Those that the client priorities become the basis for the client's goals, and most likely will be the ones the client and occupational therapist target first for further evaluation and as a focus of intervention.

Our awareness that the client has problems of occupational performance can come from ***three main sources***. First, we may be alerted to problems of occupational performance by the ***person's self-report*** that he or she is experiencing problems performing daily life tasks (e.g., via unstructured interview, COPM). Second, we may be alerted to problems of occupational performance by a ***report from others within the client constellation*** who have expressed concern about their own or the person's occupational performances (e.g., caregivers, teachers, family members who have concerns with occupational performance in relation to the person referred to occupational therapy). Third, we may be alerted to potential problems — ***discrepancies between reports*** from either various members of the client constellation (e.g., a person who says, "I have no problem," and a spouse who says, "I need to help him."), or between the client and others who are outside the client constellation (e.g., a client who reports that the person is unable to perform a task without help, and a nurse who says, "He has no problem."). These latter become *potential problems* because it is unclear whose report is more accurate.

In most cases, ***I do not recommend that the occupational therapist add to the list of potential problems by also including those task performances that we suspect may develop over time; or those we suspect may be present, but which were not discussed or were denied by the client.*** First, these potential problems are not among those reported by the client, and ***if we choose to add them, we risk losing our client-centered focus***. Moreover, most clients have sufficient self-reported problems without the need to add further any task performances we may suspect are problems.

For example, when Kristin talked with Bill about his morning routine, she was struck by a potential discrepancy. On the one hand, Bill had said that he has fallen several time in his shower and must, therefore, sit on a bench or hold onto grab bars when standing and walking in his bathroom. He also reported that putting on and taking off his shoes and socks is a problem as he has difficulty reaching his feet. On the other hand, when she asked him about putting on his trousers, he denied any problems. Kristin suspected that there may be more to this situation than she could discern at this time. Yet, she retained her client-centered focus, and reported only those tasks Bill reported were a problem. More specifically, when she documented Bill's reported strengths and problems, she was careful to indicate that it was his report, not her judgment:

> *Bill reports that he showers independently using a hand-held shower head, and while seated on a shower bench. He is able to put on his shoes and socks, but reports fatigue and physical effort. Otherwise, he reports that he is able to dress safely and independently.*

Kristin also told Bill that if at any time, any other problems emerge, he should feel free to mention them. She was also aware that after they had had a chance to work together, and they had developed greater trust and rapport, he might feel more open to mentioning dressing as a problem and/or she could again bring up the issue. If, however, he continued to report that he has no problem, and no one else in the client constellation reports a problem, ***she was prepared to "let go" of her own concerns and respect the rights and wishes of Bill, her client.***

It is important to also stress that ***as the occupational therapist summarizes the client's reported strengths, problems, and potential problems of occupational performance***, and which problems the client wants to prioritize, the occupational therapist does not include aspects of the client-centered performance context that were resources or limitations. The occupational therapist has already done that — the key elements of what we learned about Bev (see Table 4) were summarized in Documentation Example 1. And, as I noted earlier, the occupational therapist will likely consider the 10 dimensions of the client-centered performance context again, in more detail, when he or she has progressed to the step of clarifying or interpreting the cause of the client's problems with occupational performance. Rather, at this step, ***we want to remain focused on occupational performances*** that require increased effort, are inefficient, are unsafe, require verbal or physical assistance to be performed, and/or are socially inappropriate — ***those tasks that the client reports support or hinder the client's role behavior, not the contextual factors that support or hinder occupational performance***.

4.8 Case Example: Bev — Identify and Prioritize Reported Strengths and Problems of Occupational Performance

After we had written a very short summary of Bev's performance context (background information and reason for referral), we were ready to focus in on and document her reported strengths and problems of occupational performance, including those task performances that she wanted to prioritize. We found that our use of the COPM helped us in this process as it helped Bev to focus in on what of her many concerns were of most importance to her. That is, Bev had mentioned many different tasks that she is unable to perform independently, but by using the COPM, it became easier for her to reflect a bit more, and self-identify that she was actually satisfied with (and realistically needed) much of the help she receives. There were, however, tasks that she wanted to perform, especially ones that she would perform when the home health aide was not present.

When we wrote this part of our documentation, we reasoned that it was not cost effective to describe all the task performances Bev had mentioned. At the same time, we wanted to capture Bev's key concerns while conveying that we had addressed a broad range of task performances, not just PADLs; we also wanted to address IADLs and her important social activities (see Documentation Example 2).

Documentation Example 2: Bev: Initial Occupational Therapy Evaluation, Part II — Reported Level of Performance and Prioritized Task Performances

Self-reported Level of Performance:

Bev reports independence and increased effort donning garments following set-up of clothing, safe and independent toileting, safe bathing with standby assistance. Also reports independence grooming, eating, watching TV, table top games, paying bills. Satisfied with assistance received from aide and homemaker.

Self-reported problems include putting on her right shoe, getting her clothes from the closet, cooking (safety risk when standing and reaching for task objects, getting dishes in and out of the oven, getting her oxygen tubing tangled in her wheelchair when cooking). Reports desire to get out more with her daughter to go shopping and to restaurants.

Priorities:

- Put on right shoe
- Retrieve garments from closet
- Stand and stir foods when cooking
- Stand and retrieve task objects from cupboards, refrigerator, and freezer
- Remove and transport hot foods from the oven
- Manage oxygen tubing during ADL tasks

4.9 Observe Client's Task Performance and Implement Performance Analyses

Once the client has prioritized what daily life tasks to target for further evaluation and possible intervention, the occupational therapist implements the first ***performance analysis***.[23] A performance analysis involves the observation and evaluation of the

[23] Hagedorn (1995, 1997) has also used the term *performance analysis* to refer to the evaluation of a person's ability to perform daily life tasks one needs and wants to perform. However, an important distinction between her application of the term and my own (Fisher, 1997, 1998) is that she indicates that performance analyses are used to identify the "performance skill deficits" that are the underlying cause of the dysfunction. That is, Hagedorn uses the term *performance skills* to refer to sensorimotor, cognitive, psychosocial, and other body functions. As I use the term *performance skills*, the focus is directly on occupational performance — the observable, learned, goal-directed actions of performance. I hold the view that "skills are practiced abilities that show deftness, dexterity, and confidence in performance; they are goal-directed actions" (Connolly & Dalgleish, 1989, p. 894), not the person's body functions. Only when we progress to the step where we *clarify or interpret the cause* do we consider the impact of a person's body functions and impairments.

quality or effectiveness of the observable, goal-directed actions that are linked together, one after another, to construct a chain of action — a task performance (see Chapter 6 for further detail). That is, it is the client's occupational skills that are evaluated. These skills (goal-directed actions) are the motor, process, and social interaction skills that are the smallest observable units of occupational performance — not the client's person factors and body functions or impairments (see the Appendix, Table 10). Kielhofner (2008, p. 103) refers to them as "discrete purposeful actions [that] can be discerned."

The goal-directed actions we call ***motor skills*** reflect the person's effectiveness (level of skill) when moving him- or herself or task objects as the person interacts with the task objects and environment during unfolding task performances. The goal-directed actions we call ***process skills*** reflect the effectiveness of the actions the person performs he or she (a) selects, interacts with, and uses task tools and materials; (b) logically carries out individual actions and steps; and (c) modifies performance when problems are encountered. The goal-directed actions we call ***social interaction skills*** reflect the maturity and appropriateness of the person's social interactions as they unfold. The motor and process skills can be observed during any task performance that involves interacting with task tools and materials. The social interaction skills can be observed when two or more people are engaged in a task performance that involves social interaction.

They are called ***performance skills*** because each person we evaluate demonstrates more or less skill when they construct their task performances, and one of the important outcomes we hope to measure after intervention is better skill in occupational performance. That is, when the occupational therapist implements performance analyses, he or she evaluates the quality of the goal-directed actions he or she observed the person perform. More specifically, we assess skill in terms of ease (physical effort), efficiency (time and space organization), safety (risk of harm to person or damage to task objects, independence, and appropriateness of social interaction. The level of skill we observe is the result of a transaction between a person, an environment, and a task (see Figure 11). Facilitating environments and easier tasks result in a person's performance being more skilled. Skill also can improve with practice.

> *Skills are practiced abilities that show deftness, dexterity, and confidence in performance; they are goal-directed actions. . . . Skill [involves] a transaction between the performer and the environment, and to understand skilled performance it is necessary to understand the nature of the [person]–environment interaction with regard to the specific context and the goal in question. Skills are*

always jointly determined by the [person], the task, and the precise environment in which the actions take place. (Connolly & Dalgleish, 1989, p. 894)

Performance analyses should not be confused with task or activity analyses, which are intended for purposes of (a) identifying the underlying impairments that limit occupational performance or (b) the inherent therapeutic value of a task for remediating those impairments (AOTA, 1993; Hagedorn, 1995, 1997; Llorens, 1993; Mosey, 1986; Trombly, 1995b, Trombly Latham, 2008b; Watson, 1997) (see Table 5; see also Section 4.13 for further discussion of the terms *task analysis* and *activity analysis*).

Table 5 Comparison Among Performance Analyses, Task Analyses, and Activity Analyses as they are Applied in the OTIPM

Type of analysis	Based on observation of doing?	Level of analysis	Interpretation
Performance analyses	Yes	Performance skills	Quality of occupational performance — what the person does and how well
Task analyses	Yes	Personal factors, body functions, and/or the environment	Cause of the person's occupational performance problems — why the person can/cannot perform the task well
Activity analysis	No, analysis of activity in the abstract	Personal factors, body functions, and/or the environment	How to modify a task to design therapeutic occupation

To implement performance analyses, we can use standardized performance analyses such as the *Assessment of Motor and Process Skills* (AMPS) (Fisher, 2006a, 2006c), *School Version of the Assessment of Motor and Process Skills* (School AMPS) (Fisher, Bryze, Hume, & Griswold, 2007), or the *Evaluation of Social Interaction* (ESI) (Fisher & Griswold, 2009). Another option is to use the motor, process, and social interaction skill descriptions in Chapter 6 and implement informal, nonstandardized observations of occupational performances. Because performance analyses are assessments of the quality and/or effectiveness of a person's occupational performance (and not body functions and impairments), the person is scored based on what is observed — the quality of the transaction between the person and the environment as he or she performs a familiar and chosen task.

It is also important to stress that while the occupational therapist can use the existing taxonomies of motor, process, and social interaction skills included in the instruments noted above (see Chapter 6), the occupational therapist is never restricted to those taxonomies. Rather, the occupational therapist may observe and evaluate the quality of any action observed. For example, the occupational therapist may observe a child playing ball or a man fishing. She may then observe the child ***throwing*** the ball, ***kicking*** the ball, or ***passing*** the ball. She may also observe the man ***casting*** the fishing line out over the water, and then gradually ***winding*** the line back onto the reel. While the motor, process, and/or social interaction skills included in Chapter 6 may well suffice, there is no reason to not use other verbs that describe the observed actions. What is more important is that the occupational therapist observes the client's goal-directed task actions, and then evaluates their quality. That is, the occupational therapist must judge if the actions were effective, or if there was a minimal, moderate, or marked problem, and then clarify what type of problem was observed (see Table 6). ***Measureable indicators are ones the occupational therapist can see, hear, or smell.*** The use of these quality indicators will become clearer when I discuss how we progress to the phase where we actually define, describe, and document the results of our performance analyses.

4.10 Case Example: Bev — Observe Client's Task Performance and Implement Performance Analyses

On our initial visit, we observed Bev perform three tasks that she had identified as problems of occupational performance — putting on her right shoe, pouring herself a glass of ice water, and reaching for clothes from her closet. Before she performed each task, we needed to establish the ***specific performance context*** *for each task. This meant that we needed to ask a few key questions to supplement the results of our initial interview so as to gather more information related to the* ***10 dimensions for each of these tasks****. For example, we needed to* *determine where she typically puts on her shoes, who might be present to help her, and what tools and materials (including adapted equipment) she might use.*

Table 6 Measureable Quality Indicators that Can Be Used During Evaluation and Documentation of a Client's Quality of Task Performance

Type of problem observed	Severity of problem observed	
	Level	**Time**
• Physical effort	• No problem	• Time
• Time and space effectiveness	• Minimal	• Duration
• Safety	• Moderate	• Frequency
• Independence	• Marked	
• Social appropriateness		
• Verbalizations of satisfaction, pain, etc.		

More specifically, after we established the ***global*** *client-centered performance context, and summarized the resources and limitations within her performance context, as well as her reported strengths and problems of occupational performance (see Chapter 1, Figure 5 and Documentation Examples 1 and 2), we decided to implement informal performance analyses of Bev putting on her right shoe, pouring herself a glass of ice water, and reaching for clothes from her closet. Before we could implement the first of these and observe Bev putting on her right shoe, we needed to cycle back up to the first step of the intervention process, build on Bev's global client-centered performance context, and establish the* ***specific*** *client-centered performance context for putting on her right shoe. Only after we knew the specific context could we be sure that we observed Bev putting on her shoe in her typical manner.*

In a similar manner, we needed to reenter the intervention process cycle for pouring a glass of ice water and reaching for her clothes from the closet. As we established the specific client-centered performance context for each subsequent task, we continued to build on all information we had previously gathered. That is, while we would be assessing more than one task at a time, we were aware that we would be cycling through the intervention process, task by task, as if Figure 5

(Chapter 1) were comprised of several overlapping layers, one for each task (see Figure 12). As the intervention process continues, and new tasks are targeted, more layers will be added.

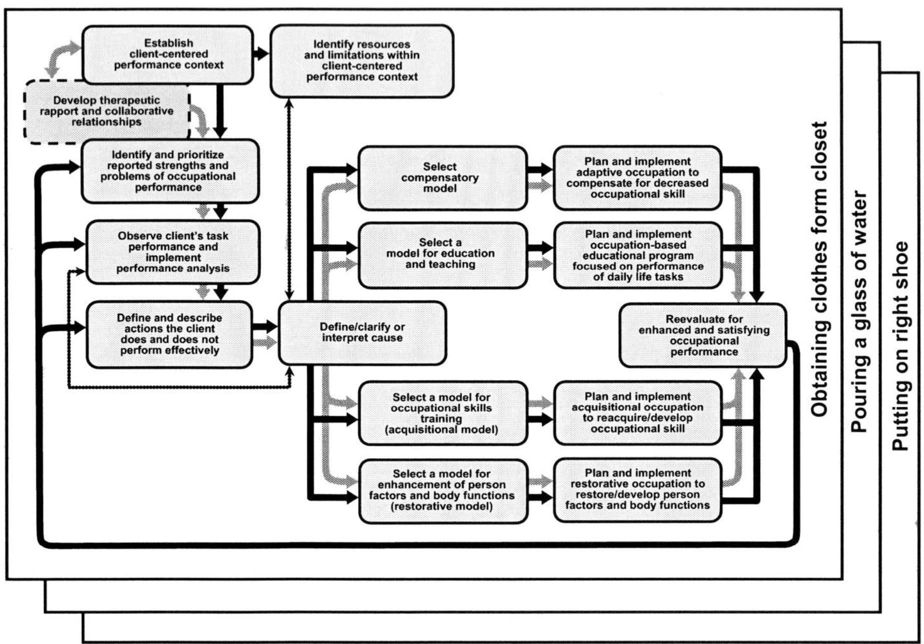

Figure 12. **Overlapping layers of the occupational therapy intervention process, one for each task addressed during Bev's initial evaluation.**

When we observed each of the three tasks, we used the motor and process skills defined in Chapter 6 as a basis for making a nonstandardized, informal evaluation of the quality of her task performances. More specifically, we noted which skills she performed effectively and which ones were characterized by increased effort (physical difficulty), decreased efficiency, safety risk, or need for assistance (see Table 6). We did not feel that an assessment of her social interaction skills was indicated.

4.11 Define and Describe Actions the Client Does and Does Not Perform Effectively

After the occupational therapist has implemented standardized or nonstandardized performance analyses, he or she is ready to *define/describe actions of performance the client did and did not perform effectively* (see Chapter 1, Figure 5). A summary of our findings must always be included in our documentation as a ***measureable baseline level of performance***. A baseline can have two forms, a global baseline and a specific baseline. The ***global baseline*** is based on the occupational therapist's observation and measureable description of the client's overall quality of task performance. The ***specific baseline*** is a more detailed, yet measurable, description of the quality of specific actions of performance that were or were not effective. To accomplish this phase of the evaluation process, I recommend that the occupational therapist ***begin with a list of actions (performance skills) that clearly were ineffective***. Then, from that list, the occupational therapist can select a subset of actions that were of most concern and which best "capture" (i.e., can be used to describe) the client's observed quality of task performance. Rarely does the number of actions included in this latter list need to be more than 10. In a similar manner, the occupational therapist may chose to select five or six actions that reflect the client's more effective actions — the client's strengths.

After the occupational therapist has prioritized up to 10 motor, process, or social interaction skills, he or she proceeds to ***group them into clusters*** of skills that have some logical relation to one another. The result of this process is usually not more than six clusters that best reflect the problems observed when the client performed prioritized daily life tasks. This step can be performed separately for each task observed, or, if the problems observed across all tasks observed are similar, the occupational therapist may choose to make just one list and set of clusters.

This step of the analysis will enable the occupational therapist to describe and clarify for the client and others the results of the occupational therapy evaluation. They will also become a source of support as the occupational therapist and the client collaborate in the process of planning interventions.

4.12 Case Example: Bev — Define and Describe the Actions of Performance the Client Does and Does Not Perform Effectively

4.12.1 Narrative Summary of Our Observations

When we observed Bev put on her right shoe, she sat in her wheelchair, placed her foot on a small footstool, and used a reacher to position the shoe in order to put her right foot into the shoe. Although she was stable when sitting in the wheelchair (Stabilizes), she experienced increased effort bending forward and using the reacher to reach for her shoe (Bends, Reaches). She experienced increased effort and inefficiency gripping and lifting her shoe (Grips, Lifts) and then placing it in the correct position to put it on (Organizes). She also experienced delays in efficiently supporting her shoe before putting it on (Handles). As a result, she had to make several attempts to position her shoe correctly (Organizes, Handles), and she needed to stop to rest five times before proceeding (Continues, Endures). Once she finally got the shoe into the correct position, she experienced increased effort sliding her foot into it (Calibrates). As she attempted to use her reacher to fasten the Velcro®[24] closures, she again had difficulty securely gripping the closures (Grips) and then exerting enough pressure to pull them tight and press them into place (Calibrates).

To pour herself a glass of ice water, Bev used her wheelchair to maneuver around in the kitchen (Walks), and then she stood to get the glass from the cupboard, ice from the freezer, and water from the sink. When she stood, she needed to hold on to the counter while opening and closing the cupboard, getting the glass from the cupboard, turning on the water at the sink, and opening the freezer and reaching in to get the ice (Stabilizes, Reaches, Moves). Preparing a glass of ice water was further complicated by her increased effort bending and reaching for objects (Bends, Reaches), making it difficult for her to open the refrigerator door even when sitting in her wheelchair (Moves). Throughout this sequence, she paused twice to rest (Endures). Finally, when she was in her wheelchair, she demonstrated increased effort moving her wheelchair, and she frequently bumped into the kitchen cabinets (Moves, Navigates).

[24] Velcro USA Inc., 406 Brown Avenue, Manchester, New Hampshire, USA, 03108.

When Bev went into her bedroom and reached for clothing from her closet (Reaches), she experienced increased effort and inefficiency moving her wheelchair into the closet and positioning herself without bumping into the doors on the closet or the objects on the floor of the closet in front of her (e.g., laundry basket) (Moves, Positions, Navigates). When she used her dressing stick to attempt to reach for and remove a pair of slacks from the rack, she again experienced increased effort bending forward, reaching up with the dressing stick, and attempting to lift the slacks from the rack (Reaches, Bends, Lifts). She paused three times to rest (Continues, Endures).

For all three tasks, Bev chose and used appropriate task objects, searched for and found them efficiently, heeded the goal, and except for her need to occasionally pause to rest, carried out the task performances without interruption (Chooses, Uses, Searches/Locates, Heeds, Continues, Endures). She demonstrated limited ability, however, to compensate for her ADL motor skill deficits and many of them persisted throughout her task performances (Accommodates, Benefits).

4.12.2 Summarizing Bev's Overall (Global) Baseline Level of Performance

After we had observed Bev and returned to the University, we first reflected on our observations and considered how to best document what we had observed. We decided to start with documenting Bev's global baseline of performance. To do this we used the quality indicators listed in Table 6, and reflected on our judgments of her overall quality of performance of each task. Our summary of Bev's global baseline is included in Part III of our Initial Note (see Documentation Example 3).

4.12.3 Creating a List of Actions of Most Concern

We then rated her performance using the motor and process skills included in the Appendix, and made a list of those that we felt reflected her ineffective task performances. We then used our professional reasoning and went back through our list and noted those that we felt best "captured" her problems with occupational performance by placing a check mark (√) beside those skills. We then added to our list those skills that best reflected Bev's most effective skills, and we marked them with an asterisk (*). Considered together, these were the skills that we felt we could use to best describe for Bev and others what we had observed. The list we made is shown in Table 7. Since the most effective and *ineffective actions we observed were rather similar across tasks, we chose to make just one list.*

4.12.4 Grouping Skills of Most Concern into Meaningful Clusters

Our next step was to group the skills we had marked into clusters that we felt were interrelated. We then wrote a short statement summarizing the key problem (or strength) reflected by the cluster. These cluster statements became the basis for our documentation of Bev's specific baseline quality of task performance. We reasoned, therefore, that it was critical that we write our statements in a form that reflected observable behavior. The following were our cluster summary statements:

- ***Cluster 1 -- Stabilizes, Reaches:*** *Bev was unstable when standing and reaching for objects from overhead cupboards. As a result, she needed to constantly hold on to the counter to prevent a fall risk.*

Table 7 Bev's Performance Skills that We Judged to Best Reflect Her Effective (*) and Ineffective (√) Quality of Task Performance

Motor skills	Process skills
Stabilizes √	Heeds *
Positions	Uses *
Reaches √	Chooses *
Bends	Handles √
Grips √	Continues
Moves √	Searches/Locates *
Lifts √	Organizes √
Walks	Navigates √
Calibrates √	Notices/Responds
Endures √	Accommodates
	Benefits

- ***Cluster 2 -- Reaches, Moves:*** *Even when seated in her wheelchair, Bev demonstrated moderate increase in physical effort moving her wheelchair close* *to her workspace (e.g., in front of the closet), and then bending forward and reaching for task objects (e.g., taps at the sink, refrigerator door, clothes hanging in closet, shoe on the floor).*

- ***Cluster 3 –- Moves, Navigates:*** *When she attempted to move her wheelchair, she frequently bumped into kitchen closets and objects in her closet.*
- ***Cluster 4 –- Lifts, Calibrates:*** *Bev also demonstrated moderate increase in effort lifting task objects (e.g., slacks from the closet, shoe from the floor), and attempting to push her foot into her shoe.*
- ***Cluster 5 –- Handles, Organizes, Grips:*** *When she used a reacher to attempt to open up her shoe and put it on, it frequently slipped out of the reacher and fell onto its side. As a result, she had to frequently reposition it.*
- ***Cluster 6 –- Endures:*** *Bev needed to pause for a rest during each of her task performances (shoes: 5 times, water: 2 times, clothes: 3 times).*

We also wanted to try to capture the idea that while Bev had many ineffective performance skills, she also had important strengths. We created, therefore, one more cluster to capture those strengths:

- ***Cluster 7 –- Heeds, Chooses, Uses, Searches/Locates:*** *Bev also demonstrated a number of strengths. For example, she consistently chose and used appropriate task objects, searched for and found them efficiently, and carried out the tasks she indicated she would perform.*

4.12.5 Summarizing Bev's Specific Baseline Level of Performance

Having created our skill clusters and summary statements, we were ready to document Bev's specific baseline level of performance. We reasoned that documenting both her global and her specific baseline level of performance would be critical, and would represent the first step of ensuring that we had documented the information we would need to evaluate the effectiveness of any interventions we implemented. To document Bev's specific baseline, we just needed to use our summary statements. We did not, however, include our final cluster related to Endures as that had already been captured in our global summary statements (see Documentation Example 3).

Documentation Example 3: Bev: Initial Occupational Therapy Evaluation, Part III — Observed Current Level of Performance

Observed Current Level of Performance

Bev was observed performing three prioritized tasks: Put on her right shoe, get a glass of ice water, and retrieve garments from her closet. The following was her baseline level of occupational performance:

Global baseline level of performance:

- Shoe: moderately inefficient and moderate increase in physical effort, from sitting using reacher, stopped to rest 5 times
- Glass of water: minimally unsafe when standing and moderate increase in physical effort; stopped to rest 2 times
- Garments from closet: moderate increase in effort, from wheelchair with dressing stick; stopped to rest 3 times

Specific baseline level of performance:

Bev was unstable when standing and reaching for objects from overhead cupboards. As a result, she needed to constantly hold on to the counter to prevent a fall risk. Even when seated in her wheelchair, Bev demonstrated moderate increase in physical effort moving her wheelchair close to her workspace (e.g., in front of the closet), and then bending forward and reaching for task objects (e.g., taps at the sink, refrigerator door, clothes hanging in closet, shoe on the floor). When she attempted to move her wheelchair, she frequently bumped into kitchen closets and objects in her closet. Bev also demonstrated moderate increase in effort lifting task objects (e.g., slacks from the closet, shoe from the floor), and attempting to push her foot into her shoe. When she used a reacher to attempt to open up her shoe and put it on, it frequently slipped out of the reacher and fell over onto its side. As a result, she had to frequently reposition it.

Bev also demonstrated a number of strengths. For example, she consistently chose and used appropriate task objects, searched for and found them efficiently, and carried out the tasks she indicated she would perform.

4.13 Define/Clarify or Interpret the Cause

After the occupational therapist has evaluated the quality of the client's performance of chosen and prioritized tasks, he or she is ready to progress to the phase of *defining/clarifying or interpreting the cause of the observed problems* (see Chapter 1, Figure 5). When we clarify the cause, we can think in terms of (a) personal factors or body function limitations, (b) physical environments, (c) social environments, and (d) societal constraints and expectations (Fisher, 1998). In fact, we could consider any aspects of the client-centered performance context that may be contributing factors to the client's ineffective occupational performance; both internal and external factors (see Tables 2 and 3, and Figure 13).

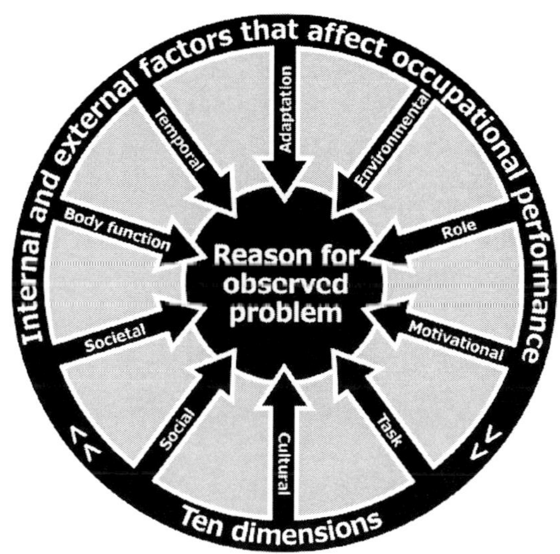

Figure 13. **Schematic diagram illustrating the 10 dimensions of the client-centered performance context in relation to the reason for the observed problem with occupational performance.**

Often, the underlying cause of a person's ineffective occupational performance is clear. When it is not, we may choose to implement further evaluations to help us to define/clarify or interpret the cause of the person's problems of occupational performance. Typically, we choose to do so when the reason for the problem is unclear and we feel that knowing the reason will impact how we might choose to intervene (e.g., determining whether a person is depressed or has poor memory, or if a person has unilateral neglect, may influence how we choose to intervene).

Determining whether a person has underlying neurologic, musculoskeletal, cognitive, and psychosocial limitations that might account for his or her problems of occupational performance can be accomplished by (a) using Figure 13 and reflecting back on the information we gathered about the ***10 dimensions*** when we established the client-centered performance context (see Table 4), (b) reflecting back on our observations of the person's occupational performances (see Section 4.12.1) and implementing ***task analyses*** (i.e., observing a person perform daily life tasks and determining the underlying cause of the person's problems of occupational performance) (see Table 5),[25] or (c) testing the person's ***discrete person factors and body functions*** (e.g., muscle stiffness, range of motion, mental status, perception, mood) and/or implementing an evaluation of the environment. In all three cases, the emphasis is on determination of what person factors, body function limitations, environmental factors, and/or sociocultural factors limit performance.

The decision as to what methods to use (e.g., reflection using the 10 dimensions shown in Figure 13, task analyses, further interview, standardized testing of person factors or body functions) and the interpretation of the results will be ***facilitated through application of principles from related knowledge and/or relevant acquisitional or restorative models***. That is, using the same rationale discussed in Section 4.1.5, the occupational therapist will likely want to link to relevant related

---

[25] Various authors have used the terms *task analysis* and/or *activity analysis* to refer to this process. ***Task analysis***, however, has been the term most commonly used to refer to the process in which ***a person is observed performing a task*** in order to identify the underlying cause of the person's limitations in occupational performance (e.g., sensorimotor, cognitive, psychosocial, motivational) (cf. Hagedorn, 1995, 1997; Watson, 1997). ***Activity analysis*** has been the term most commonly used to refer to a process in which a ***task is analyzed in isolation of the person or the observation of his or her task performance*** to (a) determine the body functions needed to perform the task, (b) identify what inherent characteristics of the task may elicit motivation or contribute to the meaningfulness of the task to a person, and (c) select, modify, and grade the task to restore underlying impairments that limit occupational performance (American Occupational Therapy Association [AOTA], 1993; Hagedorn, 1995; 1997; Llorens, 1993; Mosey, 1986; Trombly, 1995b; Watson, 1997).

More recently, this trend has been changing, but determination of which terms are used to refer to which process remains unclear. For example, Crepeau and Schell (2009) use yet another term, *occupational analysis*, to refer to an in-depth analysis of a person's occupations and their meanings, but they continue to use the term *activity analysis* in a manner similar to that discussed above. Moreover, Trombly-Latham (2008a) sometimes uses the term *activity analysis* to refer to both performance analyses and activity analyses: "Activity analysis is used to analyze and assess performance [performance analysis], to select occupations to remediate deficient capacities and abilities, or, knowing the person's skills, abilities, and capacities, to select and modify activity to ensure successful completion of the activity" [activity analysis] (p. 2). Yet elsewhere, she indicates that *activity analysis* and *task analysis* can be viewed as synonyms, but that the latter pertains primarily to work assessments (Trombly Latham, 2008b).

To further complicate the situation, while Trombly Latham (2008b) cites Fisher (1998), she goes on the say that "both activity and performance analyses entail unnesting the components of tasks [global PADLs and IADLs, e.g., meal preparation] and activities [smaller, chosen units of PADLs and IADLs, e.g., grilling fish] that constitute occupation and determining what abilities, skills, and capacities are needed to do the specified activity or that may improve if the person does that activity" (p. 363). Even if she had retained a focus only on performance skills, misunderstanding arises because Fisher (1998), specified that performance analyses are used to evaluate the quality of a person's occupational performance, ***not*** to determine what underlying capacities are needed to perform the task.

knowledge (e.g., anthropology, neuroscience, psychology) and/or restorative or acquisitional models (e.g., social, biomechanical, developmental, Model of Human Occupation, sensory integration) to help us better understand the basis of the person's problems of occupational performance.

It is also at this point that the occupational therapist may choose to implement formal or informal evaluations of the environment. Again, the occupational therapist may choose to link to other selected practice models, such as the Model of Human Occupation (Kielhofner, 2008). A wide range of environmental assessments also are available (Letts et al., 1994).

4.13.1 Clarifying the Cause Within the True Top–down Reasoning Framework of the OTIPM (versus a Top–to–bottom–up Framework)

A unique feature of the OTIPM is that the occupational therapist is encouraged to follow a step-by-step, true top–down professional reasoning process to determine what are the client's strengths and problems of occupational performance before clarifying the cause of the client's problems of occupational performance. That is, we begin by first determining what tasks are identified by the client as strengths or problems of occupational performance. Then, rather than jumping immediately to implementing task analyses (i.e., determining what person factors or body functions, environmental factors, and/or societal constraints or expectations might be the underlying cause of the client's problem), we first implement performance analyses to determine what specific goal-directed actions of each task performance are or are not problems for the client (see Chapter 1, Figures 1 and 3, and Table 5). This enables us to focus our subsequent evaluation and intervention procedures on those goal-directed actions that are most limiting the quality of the person's occupational performance while building on those that are strengths. Our ultimate goal will be to design and implement interventions to restore or compensate for Bev's ineffective actions.

In this way, the OTIPM is unlike other so-called top–down frameworks that actually follow a top–to–bottom–up reasoning process (see Chapter 1, Section 1.2.3). When using top–to–bottom–up models (e.g., CAOT, 2002; Kielhofner, 2008; Trombly Latham, 2008a), the occupational therapist more commonly begins by establishing the client's performance context, and possibly, strengths and problems of occupational performance, but then jumps to implementing task analyses to determine the underlying cause of the client's problem (see Chapter 1, Figure 3). By omitting the process of implementing a performance analysis and defining the actions of performance that the person does and does not perform effectively, top–to–bottom–up models attempt to directly link reported levels of occupational performance to underlying impairments and person factors and body functions (and sometimes, but less often, features of the environment). Yet, as I discussed earlier in Chapter 1, Section 1.2.2, ***research has not demonstrated a strong enough relationship between these underlying factors and ADL performance to be able to make valid predictions*** about why a person may be experiencing problems with occupational performance (Bernspång, Asplund, Eriksson, & Fugl-Meyer, 1987; Jongbloed, Brighton, & Stacey, 1988; Judge, Schechtman, Cress, & the FICSIT Group, 1996; Lichtenberg & Nanna, 1994; Pincus et al., 1989; Reed, Jagust, & Seab, 1989; Skurla, Rogers, & Sunderland, 1988; Teri, Borson, Kiyak, & Yamagishi, 1989).[26]

An added advantage of using the true top–down approach of the OTIPM is that, ***after*** we implement performance analyses and define/describe the actions of performance the person does and does not perform effectively, we still can readily link to various restorative practice models and implement ***task analyses*** based on the very same performances we observed when we implemented performance analyses (see lower dotted line in Figure 5, Chapter 1). The result is more thorough, but cost-effective, assessment because (a) the occupational therapist remains more focused on the client's concerns (something that also can be achieved in any model that stresses a client-centered approach), (b) invalid inferences are avoided, and (c) time-consuming and unnecessary testing of discrete underlying factors is prevented.

4.14 Case Example: Bev — Define/Clarify or Interpret the Cause

When we considered the cause of Bev's observed problems with occupational performance, we reflected both on the 10 dimensions shown in Figure 13 and back on our observations of her task performances, and readily identified body function limitations and environmental factors that most affected her occupational performances. As part of this process, we implemented a task analysis by linking to the biomechanical model — it was clear to us that her limited strength and physical endurance were limiting her occupational performances; her limitations in range of motion in her right hip and knee were secondary. We did not feel that there was any reason to administer additional evaluations associated with the biomechanical model to assess her range of motion, strength, or endurance (Flinn,

[26] The references I have included here represent only selected examples from different areas of practice. We all must assume responsibility to implement literature searches and reviews to determine what evidence exists for the methods we use.

Trombly Latham, & Podolski, 2008; Greene & Roberts, 2005). Such procedures are costly in terms of time, and would yield little information beyond what we already knew. Said another way, we reasoned that knowing that Bev had 90 or 110 degrees of movement, fair or good muscle strength, or could complete a given number of repetitions of a movement in a given unit of time would not help us to determine what were her problems of occupational performance nor how to intervene.

While one of the major reasons for Bev's limitations in occupational performance was her limited activity tolerance (e.g., decreased strength and endurance in the context of ADL task performances), there also appeared to be several features of the physical environment that were hindering the quality of her occupational performance. That is, by implementing another task analysis based on principles derived from the Model of Human Occupation (Kielhofner, 2008), we identified a number of environmental demands and constraints associated with the spaces and objects in Bev's apartment. Her apartment was small and had limited storage space. As a result, Bev had to store items on the kitchen counters and on the floor of the closet. The closet door also constrained her ability to access the closet, and the clothes rack in her closet was too high for Bev to easily reach her clothes. Another environmental constraint was the design of Bev's shoes which did not facilitate her getting them on.

Societal constraints further added to the causes of Bev's problems. Her limited financial resources would prevent her from moving to a larger apartment, making major modifications to her present apartment, or purchasing new shoes. In Bev's case, her motivation and her social environment were supports rather than causes of her problems of occupational performance. A summary of our conclusions is shown in Documentation Example 4.

Documentation Example 4: Bev: Initial Occupational Therapy Evaluation, Part IV — Interpretation of Cause

Interpretation

Cognition, memory, and judgment appear intact. Frailty, low activity tolerance, and decreased trunk mobility/range of motion limit quality of ADL task performance. Small rooms, limited space, and closet design further hinder ADL task performance.

4.15 Document Client's Baseline and Goals

In order to evaluate if a client has improved following occupational therapy intervention, it is essential that the occupational therapist document the client's baseline and goals in a manner that is observable and measurable. Both must be accomplished before progressing to the implementation of any intervention. In a similar manner, new observable and measureable baselines (i.e., reevaluation baselines) and new goals must also be documented, if relevant, during the ongoing intervention process. Documentation of measurable baselines, goals, and, later in the process, the intervention results provide the basis for gathering the critically needed evidence that our interventions are or are not effective. ***Systematically documenting the effectiveness of our interventions also provides us with an important foundation for communicating to others our unique role, and demonstrating that our focus is on occupation — the person's ability to perform needed and desired daily life tasks.***

As discussed in Section 4.11, the client's baseline level of performance is a summary if the client's observed quality of task performance. Again, the baseline can be written as a global baseline and/or a specific baseline. Each baseline should include a description of (a) what the person did (what task the person performed), and (b) how well the person performed the task (the quality of performance, based on the quality indicators in Table 6).

Formulation of a client-centered goal requires that the occupational therapist collaborate with the client in the process of determining the client's next higher level of performance. If the client is a ***person who is unable to communicate***, it is critical that we work together with others who know the client (e.g., family members) and who can best articulate what they believe the client would want. Likewise, when we work with ***clients who can communicate, but who experience difficulty articulating clear or realistic goals***, we must commit to working collaboratively with our clients and assist them in the process of identifying clear, measurable, and realistic goals — ones that the client wants to achieve, ***not*** ones we select for the client.

When we document the client's goals, we again use the quality indicators listed in Table 6. It is also important that we do not include our planned interventions in the goals. Instead, we describe what the client will do. Our planned interventions are documented in the intervention plan. ***The minimally required components of a goal include (a) what task the client will perform, and (b) how well the client will perform it.*** Other recommended components are shown in Table 8.

Table 8 Components of Baseline, Goal, and New (Reevaluation) Baseline Statements

Baseline and reevaluation statements

- ***Who*** performed the task
- ***What*** did the client do (task)
- ***How*** well did the client do what the client did (quality indicators)

Goal statements

- ***Who*** will perform the task
- ***What*** will the client be able to do following intervention (task)
- ***How*** well will the client do what the client anticipates being able to do (quality indicators)
- ***When*** will the client have reached the goal

When we document the client's goals, it is important to keep in mind that most clients do not have experience formulating or writing goals. Often, therefore, it is the occupational therapist who actually formulates and writes the goal. In this process, however, ***the occupational therapist must work closely with the person and others in the client constellation to formulate goals that are realistic, but consistent with the client's intentions and desires***, while ensuring that they are written in a manner that is occupation-focused, observable, and measurable.

4.16 Case Example: Bev — Document the Client's Goals

When we met with Bev, she seemed quite clear as to what were her goals. To ensure no misunderstanding, however, we confirmed with her that we had correctly understood what she wanted to be able to do so that what we wrote in our report would accurately reflect her intentions. For example, she wanted to be able to get her clothes from the closet, and she did not want "it to be so hard." We then reviewed with her what we had observed — she had demonstrated a moderate increase in effort, she performed the task from wheelchair, she used a dressing stick to reach for and lift her slacks, and she stopped to three times to rest — and asked her, "What would you like to be different?" Through more discussion, with us asking her questions and Bev clarifying (e.g., Do you want to do it standing, or is it okay to sit in your wheelchair? How do you feel about your need to take a rest?"). Through this collaborative process, with us asking guiding questions, and Bev determining what was and was not acceptable, we worked together to formulate Bev's goals. She preferred to formulate short term goals, focusing on what she might be able to do after only one or two occupational therapy sessions. Respecting her wishes, that is what we did. We included Bev's goals in our documentation (see Documentation Example 5).

Documentation Example 5: Bev: Client's Goals

Goals

- Bev will don her right shoe independently, demonstrating only minimal increase in physical effort, stopping to rest no more than three times
- Bev will retrieve garments from her closet independently, demonstrating only minimal increase in physical effort, stopping to rest no more than once
- Bev will stand and retrieve objects from cupboards, refrigerator, and freezer safely, demonstrating only minimal increase in physical effort and stopping to rest no more than one time.
- Bev will manage oxygen tubing efficiently, without it getting tangled in wheelchair

4.17 Select Intervention Model and Plan and Implement Occupation-based Interventions

Once the occupational therapist has completed the initial evaluation, and collaborated with the client to formulate client-centered goals, he or she is ready to select one or more intervention models (see Chapter 1, Figure 5). We ***select restorative models*** when we judge, based on existing evidence, that development or restoration of person factors and body functions through engagement in occupation will likely result in the development or restoration of effective person factors and body functions during occupational performance. We ***select acquisitional models*** when we judge, based on existing evidence, that development or reacquisition of occupation skill through engagement in occupation will likely result in more effective occupational performance. We ***select the compensatory model*** **and/*****or acquisitional models*** if (a) restoration of person factors and body functions are unlikely to improve or result in enhance occupational performance, (b) restoration would take more time, effort, or money than we have available (Trombly, 1993); or (c) there are societal directives (e.g., legislation) to focus on occupational performance and role competence. Finally, we select ***only the compensatory model*** if neither restorative methods nor acquisitional occupational skills training are likely to result in enhanced occupational performance, and/or time constraints limit the feasibility of other options. It is also important to point out that the occupational therapist may choose to use all three (and/or perhaps even an education and teaching model if he or she plans to implement client workshops or seminars), again with the caveat that the ***use of any model should be based on available evidence that it will likely result in improved occupational performance***.

When planning intervention, and determining what model(s) to use, the occupational therapist can also reflect on the 10 dimensions of the client-centered performance context, and systematically determine what changes are most likely to result in desired outcomes following intervention (see Figure 14). For example, the occupational therapist can consider if changes in the environment or the client's body functions are most likely to be effective. Moreover, in designing effective interventions, the occupational therapist can consider if motivation, role behavior, cultural differences or issues, and so on need to be addressed.

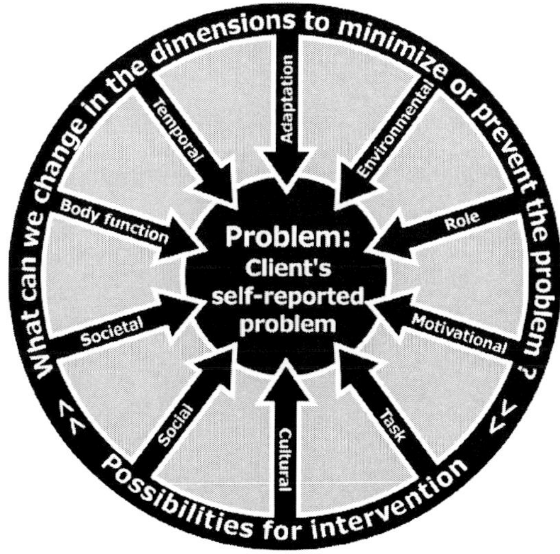

Figure 14. **Schematic diagram illustrating the 10 dimensions of the client-centered performance context in relation to considering what changes to make as part of planned interventions.**

4.18 Case Example: Bev — Select Intervention Models and Plan and Implement Occupation-based Interventions

4.18.1 Case Example: Bev — Session 1, Planning Restorative Occupation to Restore Body Functions and Acquisitional Occupation to Reacquire Occupational Skill

Given that Bev's goals included donning her right shoe, retrieving clothes from her closet, and retrieving objects from cupboards and the refrigerator, we discussed with Bev at the end of our initial visit a variety of options for what she could do during her second occupational therapy session. That is, after we, together with Bev, reflected back on Bev's baseline and goals, and her prognosis for change, we shared with her the idea that we could use a combination of an occupation-based restorative model and an occupation-based acquisitional model, and collaborate with Bev to engage her in (a) ***restorative occupation*** *to enhance her activity tolerance, and (b)* ***acquisitional occupation*** *to restore more effective actions. That is, we suggested that we could give Bev the opportunity to practice getting dressed and/or standing and reaching for objects in her kitchen or for clothes in her closet (from her wheelchair). We also shared with her our reasoning that engagement in chosen occupations that would require her to perform activity over longer and longer periods of time likely would help her to build up her activity tolerance and, at the same time, develop greater occupational skill (see Chapter 2, Figure 8). We also discussed the possibilities for progressively grading her engagement in PADL and IADL tasks as her activity tolerance and/or occupational skill improved in the future.*

Bev agreed with our proposed plan, and chose to carry out the PADL task of total body dressing and the IADL task of pouring herself a glass of milk during her next occupational therapy session. We realized that her performance of these two tasks would have an added benefit that we had not anticipated — it would enable us to also carry out a ***standardized performance analysis*** *using the AMPS (Fisher, 2006a, 2006b, 2006c). Hence, we could implement cost-effective occupational therapy by combining intervention with assessment. We included our intervention plan in our documentation of our initial visit (see Documentation Example 6).*

Documentation Example 6: Bev: Intervention Plan

Intervention Plan
• AMPS evaluation • Graded restorative occupation to increase activity tolerance • Occupational skills training • Adaptation (modify environment, provide adapted equipment, teach compensatory strategies) • Collaborative consultation and education

During the week that ensued between our visits, the students and I discussed appropriate restorative and acquisitional models to use with Bev as we planned and simultaneously implemented restorative and acquisitional occupation designed to enable Bev to improve her activity tolerance and reacquire some effective actions (i.e., occupational skill) (see Chapter 2, Figure 8). More specifically, we reasoned that since Bev's primary body function limitations were related to her poor strength and endurance, we could select the biomechanical model (Flinn, Jackson, Gray, & Zemke, 2008; Greene & Roberts, 2005) from among the many restorative models we had available to us. We could then apply principles of activity analysis and synthesis (AOTA, 1993; Mosey, 1986) to Bev's chosen activities to plan and implement appropriate interventions. We also reasoned that if she practiced those daily occupations of importance to her, we could apply principles of acquisition derived from yet other models, including behavioral and learning models (Bruce & Borg, 2002; Mosey, 1986). In both cases, as her activity tolerance increased and her actions became more effective, we could progressively grade her occupations so that the demands of the tasks would increase as she improved.

4.18.2 Case Example: Bev — Session 2, Implementing a Standardized AMPS Performance Analysis and Observing Bev Perform Two ADL Tasks

Before we could engage Bev in restorative and acquisitional occupation, and simultaneously implement a standardized AMPS performance analysis,[27] *we had to*

[27] ***The AMPS is a standardized test of participation and/or complex activity*** (ADL ability) as defined by the World Health Organization (WHO, 2001). This is in contrast to the common misconception that the AMPS is an assessment of impairments and body function limitations (see the Appendix, Table 10). It is

establish the specific client-centered performance context *for the two tasks she was to perform. This required that we briefly interview her to determine such things as where she typically performed these tasks, and what tools and materials she usually uses (e.g., Does she sit in her wheelchair or use her walker? Does she use a reacher or dressing stick? What clothes would she put on? Where does she store the glassware and the milk?).*

We then ensured that the task environment was set up as Bev typically would have it, and observed her get dressed and then pour herself a glass of milk. After we had observed her perform each AMPS task, we returned to the university and scored her quality of performance on each of the 16 ADL motor and 20 ADL process skills included in the AMPS, once for each task performed.

When we were done rating her quality of performance of each AMPS task, we again defined/described the actions that Bev did and did not perform effectively, and created summary clusters of the skills most reflecting her quality of occupational performance. When she performed the task of pouring herself a glass of milk, her overall performance was very similar to what we had observed when she poured herself a glass of ice water the week before. Her performance during dressing, however, revealed a number of problems that we had not been able to identify when she merely put on her right shoe and reached for clothes from the closet.

More specifically, Bev again demonstrated moderate increase in physical effort and inefficiency moving her wheelchair into her closet and positioning herself without bumping into the right closet door. She demonstrated marked increase in physical effort when she bent forward and reached for her clothes from the closet with her dressing stick and when she used her reacher to reach down to put on her right sock and shoe. She was also markedly inefficient as she required repeated trials to hook the hanger with the dressing stick. Moreover, when she started to lift the hanger off of the clothes rack, the hanger was not well supported on the end of the dressing stick. As a result, she dropped her slacks onto the laundry basket on the floor of her closet. She also demonstrated moderate increase in physical effort and inefficiency pulling up her slacks and her socks. She again was very inefficient organizing her right shoe to put it on. By this time, she had become extremely fatigued. She had stopped many times to rest and her

probable that this confusion has occurred because the names of some of the AMPS skill items (e.g., Stabilizes, Attends, Sequences) are similar to terms we might use to describe physical and cognitive impairments and body function limitations (e.g., poor balance, attentional deficits, poor sequencing abilities) (see Fisher, 2006b for more detail).

pace had slowed considerably. She required assistance, therefore, to put on her shoes and fasten them. In the context of performing a task that required greater activity tolerance, Bev was unable to compensate for her persistent problems.

4.18.3 Case Example: Bev — Session 2, Defining/Clarifying Cause

Having implemented two standardized performance analyses (AMPS observations) and defined/described the actions that Bev did not perform effectively, we now needed to define/clarify or interpret the cause of her problems with those tasks. As her performance when pouring herself a glass of milk was so similar to when she had prepared herself a glass of ice water, we had no new information to add to what we already had reported. We also recognized that we would learn more about her cooking skills when we had a chance to further assess her ability to stand and stir foods and manage hot foods from the oven.

In contrast, even before we returned to the university to score her quality of performance, we realized that her marked increase in physical effort with the dressing task was likely due to Bev's underlying limitations in strength and endurance that, in turn, were limiting her activity tolerance. We were also able to confirm that the right closet door, the clothes rack, and the design of her shoes were environmental factors that were having a profound effect on her performance. This led us, toward the end of our second visit, to revise of our intervention plan, select the compensatory model, and begin to plan and implement adaptive occupations to compensate for Bev's ineffective actions during total body dressing (see Chapter 2, Figure 9).

4.18.4 Case Example: Bev — Session 2, Selecting and Implementing Adaptive Occupation to Compensate for Ineffective Actions

Collaborative Consultative, Education, and Adaptation

Before we began to implement adaptive occupation based on the compensatory model, we asked Bev about her perceived experience of difficulty and shared with her our perceptions of the quality of her performance and the cause of her problems. This meant that we built on the therapeutic rapport/collaborative relationship between Bev and ourselves that had been developing since we first met Bev and began to establish the client-centered performance context (see the lighter grey arrows in Figure 5, Chapter 1).

She expressed a great deal concern with her performance. "I get so tired. It is hard. I wish it was easier." She was also aware that the physical environment only contributed to her becoming very tired. "Look where I'm living and the space I have. It is a good thing I've had a good attitude." Her concerns and insights confirmed for us the need to revise our intervention plan and start implementing adaptive occupation to enable her to compensate for those ineffective actions that could not be restored and/or those occupational skills that could not be reacquired (see Chapter 2, Figure 9).

We, therefore, began to plan and implement adaptive occupation by talking to her about the possibility of removing the right door on her closet and lowering the rack in her closet so that she could more easily access her clothes. Her initial reaction was one of hesitation. We were not sure if she was somewhat resistant to the idea of "change" or more concerned about what options would be acceptable to the apartment management. As we probed further, the latter seemed to be the issue. We also were alert to the fact that, with her limited financial resources, she might be concerned about the cost of making modifications to her apartment.

Clearly, we needed to ***extend our consultative partnership to include other persons who were not members of the client constellation****, but who had access to needed information or who would be impacted by the proposed changes. As we talked with Bev, we learned the name of the apartment manager, who was the person she thought we would need to contact regarding permission to remove the right door and install a new rack in her closet. Bev supported our consulting with the apartment manager to determine if we could implement our recommended changes, and, if so, how the manager would prefer we proceed. Bev expressed concern, however, about the potential cost of a new clothes rack.*

We felt it important, therefore, to extend the consultative partnerships to include not only the apartment manager, but also Bev's daughter. It was her daughter who had originally referred Bev to us. We asked Bev if she thought that her daughter might be able to provide her mother with the financial support needed to buy a new clothes rack, and how Bev would feel about that. As we proceeded to talk to Bev about her shoes, it was clear that Bev felt that her daughter would be the person who should talk to the physical therapist or orthotist about the possibility of modifying Bev's shoes so that they would be easier for Bev to put on. We developed, therefore, a plan with Bev whereby we would contact both the apartment manager and her daughter early the next week.

Once the members of the consultative partnership were identified, the next step was for us to simultaneously implement methods of ***collaborative consultation*** *(Fisher, 1997, 2002/2006),* ***education*** *(teaching-learning) (Mosey, 1986; Trombly, 1995c), and* ***adaptation*** *(Fisher, 1997, 2002/2006; Trombly 1995c) (see also Chapter 2, Figure 9 and Chapter 3, Section 3.2.2). We were aware that what the occupational therapist commonly does at this phase is to build on the newly developed and extended collaborative relationships, and work together with the members of the consultative partnership to propose and develop strategies for intervention based on the principles of adaptation. That is, the members of the collaborative partnership need to work together to establish mutually-acceptable strategies for achieving the client's goals (e.g., ones that both the client and the caregiver can agree on).*

In Bev's case, the emphasis was on consultation and adaptation; the demands for education were minimal.[28] *For example, we would want to consult with the apartment manager regarding the removal of Bev's right closet door and the installation of the clothes rack, at a height Bev could more easily reach. If the apartment manager agreed to these ideas, all of us would need to collaborate on developing a plan for implementing them. For example, we would need to provide instruction to whomever was to purchase the rack (probably her daughter) as to what size and type of rack she should purchase (e.g., the rack should have a shelf where Bev could store some of the things currently on the floor of her closet). We would also need to collaborate on developing a plan to provide instruction to whomever was to install the rack (either her daughter or an employee of the apartment complex) about the correct placement of the rack in Bev's closet.*

Adaptation Strategies

As I noted earlier, adaptation includes providing adapted equipment or assistive technology, teaching the client alternative strategies or compensatory techniques, and modifying the task or the physical or social environment (see Chapter 2, Figure 9). For occupational therapists, who are experts in adaptation, the list of possibilities is endless. In Bev's case, the adaptations we considered to

[28] More clear examples of education might include teaching a caregiver in how to (a) safely transfer a person who has had a stroke, or (b) cue a person with dementia. Another example would be teaching a child with cerebral palsy how to use his new adapted communication board. In the compensatory model, education is applied to the various members of the consultative partnership responsible for implementing the interventions — whether it is training the client how to perform the task given environmental modifications or the provision of adapted equipment or assistive technology, or it is training a caregiver or service extender to provide physical or verbal assistance.

help her overcome her ineffective actions while dressing were removing the door from her closet, installing a new rack in her closet, and proposing modifications to her shoes — all examples of modifications of the physical environment.

4.18.5 Case Example: Bev —Planning and Implementing Ongoing Intervention

Clarify the Intervention Plan for the Next Week

At the end of Bev's second visit, we had not only developed a plan to implement adaptive occupation related to her dressing, we also collaborated with her to develop a plan for continued implementation of restorative occupation. More specifically, we talked with Bev about preparing a meal that would involve her stirring food at the counter or stove and removing hot pans from the oven. The task she chose to perform the next week was a dish she called "taco lasagna." Observing her prepare taco lasagna would allow us to (a) implement nonstandardized performance analyses of her identified priorities of stirring food and managing hot pans, (b) continue her participation in restorative occupations designed to increase her activity tolerance, and (c) continue implementing adaptive occupation (collaborative consultation, education, and adaptation), as needed, related to her cooking skills, per our revised intervention plan. Before we left, we also suggested to Bev that at our next visit we could plan share with her the results of our AMPS observation, and then discuss, in more detail, ideas for further intervention.

As part of preparing to share with her the results of our AMPS observation, we scored her quality of ADL task performance using the standardized criteria in the AMPS manual (Fisher, 2006c), created a list of skills of most concern, grouped them into clusters, wrote summary statements, interpreted the cause of her observed problems with ADL task performance (see Sections 4.18.2 and 4.18.3), and then documented Bev's second visit in a progress note (see Documentation Example 7). Again, as with her initial note, our emphasis was on Bev's occupational performances and not person factors and body functions or the underlying cause of her difficulties. Her computer-generated AMPS Narrative Report is shown in Documentation Example 8 and her computer-generated AMPS Graphic Report is shown in Documentation Example 9.

Documentation Example 7: Bev: Progress Note (SOAP Note, for Session 2)

Progress Note

S: "I get so tired. It is hard. I wish it was easier." "Look where I am living and the space I have. It is a good thing I've had a good attitude."

O: Bev seen this date for restorative occupation to increase activity tolerance, occupational skills training related to ADL, collaborative consultation regarding adaptive/compensatory strategies, and administration of the Assessment of Motor and Process Skills (AMPS). Bev performed two AMPS tasks of her choice and that she prioritized for intervention: Total body dressing and Beverage from the refrigerator. AMPS Narrative Report (Documentation Example 8) and AMPS Graphic Report (Documentation Example 9) placed in chart.

A: During task of getting dressed, Bev demonstrated marked increase in physical effort, especially as she bent forward and reached for her clothes from her closet and when putting on her right shoe and sock. Her performance was markedly inefficient (e.g., frequent interruptions, organizing task objects in workspace). Her performance was slow and she had to stop frequently to rest. She needed occasional physical assistance to complete the task due to fatigue.

When getting a beverage from the refrigerator, Bev demonstrated moderate increase in physical effort and was minimally unsafe when standing to reach for objects from cupboards and refrigerator. Bev's difficulties compensating for her ADL motor and ADL process skill deficits indicate implementation of adaptive occupation is indicated. Refer to AMPS report for more information.

P: Consult with apartment manager to discuss removing closet door and installing a lower clothes rack in closet. Consult with daughter to discus options for modifying Bev's shoes. Assess priorities 3 and 5 from initial evaluation (see Documentation Example 2. Continue, as tolerated, per intervention plan.

Documentation Example 8: Bev's Computer-generated AMPS Narrative Report (for Session 2)

OCCUPATIONAL THERAPY EVALUATION OF ADL ABILITY

Results and Interpretation of an Assessment of Motor and Process Skills (AMPS) Evaluation

Therapist: Anne G. Fisher
Client: Bev M
Age: 65

AMPS EVALUATION
The Assessment of Motor and Process Skills (AMPS) was administered to Bev M as a means of evaluating her ability to perform activities of daily living (ADL) tasks. As part of the AMPS assessment, the occupational therapist conducted an interview to gain a better understanding of the everyday tasks (occupations) that have been presenting a challenge for her, as well as those everyday tasks that she has been performing with little difficulty. She was offered a choice of familiar and relevant tasks that she had identified as presenting problems in everyday life. She chose to perform 2 of the tasks that were offered: "Upper and lower body dressing - garments stored", and "Beverage from the refrigerator." When the AMPS was administered, the occupational therapist assessed the amount of effort, independence, efficiency, and safety that she exhibited during the performance of these tasks.

OVERALL QUALITY OF PERFORMANCE
Bev showed evidence of minimal safety risk, markedly effortful, and markedly inefficient ADL task performance and she needed occasional assistance to complete the 2 ADL tasks.

SPECIFIC SKILLS THAT MOST IMPACTED PERFORMANCE
More specifically, Bev's performance of the above noted ADL tasks was limited by:

- Momentarily losing balance and/or needing to support herself on external objects while moving through the environment or interacting with task objects (Stabilizes)
- Increased effort when reaching for or placing task objects (Reaches)
- Increased effort bending to sit down or stand up (Bends)
- Difficulty completing tasks without obvious evidence of physical fatigue (Endures)
- Failing to maintain a consistent and effective rate of task performance (Paces)
- Pausing during actions or task steps, delaying task progression (Continues)
- Organizing workspaces so that they are too crowded and/or too spread out and difficulty spatially arranging clothing (Organizes)
- Decreased skill accommodating for and preventing problems from occurring, and problems persisted or recurred during task performances (Accommodates and Benefits)

OVERALL ADL MOTOR ABILITY
ADL motor ability is an overall measure of a person's observed skill when moving oneself or task objects as needed for ADL task performance. Bev's ADL motor ability measure of -0.44 logit is plotted in relationship to the AMPS motor cutoff measure on the AMPS Graphic Report. Her ADL motor ability is below the AMPS motor cutoff. This indicates that she has increased effort when she performs ADL tasks. To put this in perspective, approximately 95% of well, healthy persons of Bev's age have ADL motor ability measures between 1.33 and 3.41 logits. This indicates that her ADL motor performance is lower than age expectations.

Documentation Example 8 (continued)

OVERALL ADL PROCESS ABILITY

ADL process ability is a global measure of a person's observed skill in efficiently (a) selecting, interacting with, and using task tools and materials; (b) carrying out individual task actions and steps; and (c) modifying task performance when problems are encountered. On the AMPS Graphic Report, Bev's ADL process ability measure of 0.24 logit is below AMPS process scale cutoff. This indicates that she is experiencing decreased safety, independence and/or efficiency when she performs familiar ADL tasks. As a basis for comparison, 95% of well, healthy persons of Bev's age have ADL process ability *measures between 0.78 and 2.62 logits, thus her ADL process ability measure is lower than age expectations.*

SUMMARY OF MAIN FINDINGS

- Bev's ADL motor and ADL process ability measures are both below the AMPS cutoffs and below age expectations, indicating that she is experiencing increased effort, decreased efficiency, decreased safety, and/or the need for assistance when performing chosen, familiar, and life relevant ADL tasks.

Occupational therapy services may be indicated to enhance and/or prevent further decline of Bev's ADL task performance.

If there are any questions regarding this evaluation, please do not hesitate to contact me.

Anne G. Fisher

Documentation Example 9: Bev's Computer-generated AMPS Graphic Report (for Session 2)

ASSESSMENT OF MOTOR AND PROCESS SKILLS (AMPS) GRAPHIC REPORT

Client:	Bev M		MOTOR	PROCESS
Occupational therapist:	Anne G. Fisher	Evaluation 1	-0.44	0.24

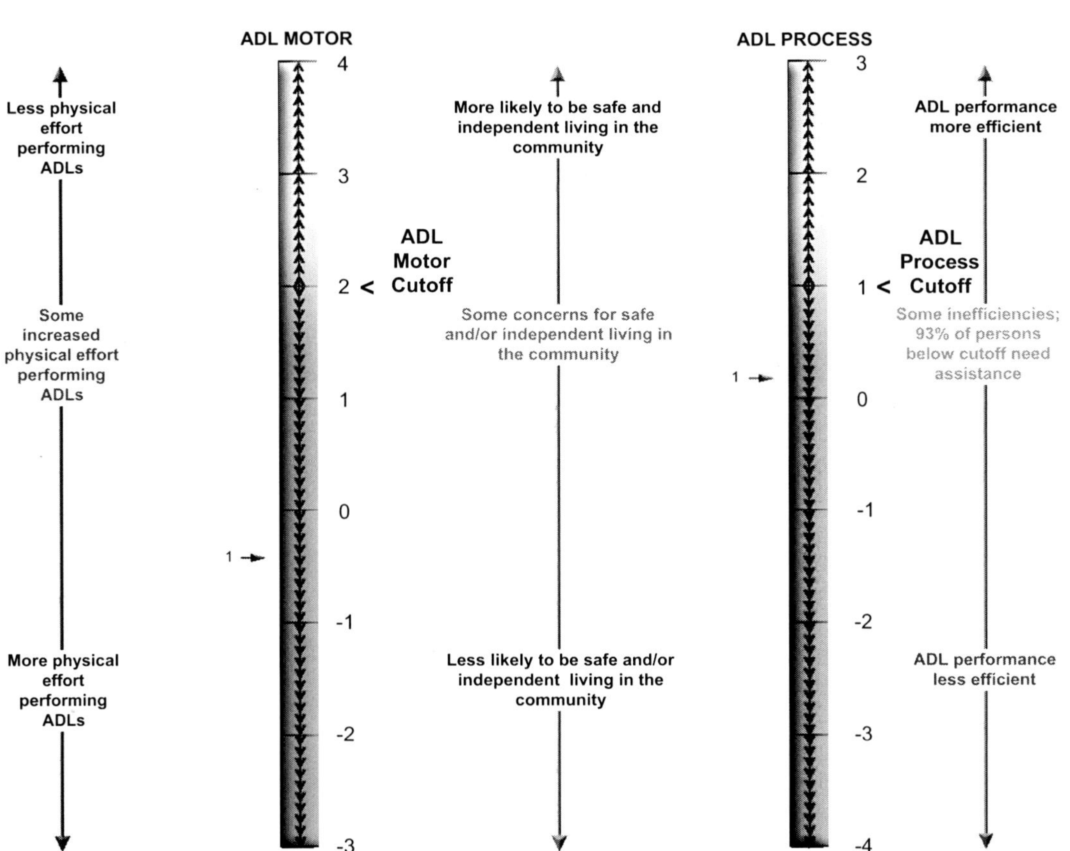

The numbers on the ADL motor and ADL process scales are units of ADL ability (logits). The results are reported as ADLmotor and ADL process measures plotted in relation to the AMPS scale cutoffs. Measures below the cutoffs indicate that there was dminished quality or effectiveness of performance of instrumental and/or personal activities of daily living (ADL). See the AMPS Narrative Report for further infomation regarding the interpretation of a single AMPS evaluation.

Bev's ADL process ability of 0.24 logit[29] *was below the AMPS process scale cutoff. Persons below the AMPS process scale cutoff are those who have a very high probability of needing assistance to live in the community (Fisher, 2006a). This supported what we knew about Bev — she did need and received assistance from others. We were also aware that we could, if needed, use this information to support any recommendations we might have related to Bev needing continued assistance in the future.*

Her ADL motor ability of -0.44 logit was quite low and well below the AMPS motor scale cutoff. Since she also had generalized ADL motor skill problems, we realized that Bev probably had limited potential to benefit from further restorative occupation. The fact that Bev's ADL process ability was near zero could further suggest that we should only introduce restorative and/or acquisitional occupation cautiously. Rather, when considered together, her ADL motor and ADL process ability measures indicated Bev's greatest potential was to benefit from the therapeutic use of adaptive occupation (Fisher, 2006a).

We realized that having the ***objective results of a standardized test like the AMPS both can support our professional reasoning, and provide us with a political tool*** *that we can use support any recommendations that we might make related to placement and intervention. Moreover, if we readminister the AMPS when we implement our reevaluation, we will be able to document objectively any improvements Bev made as a result of our interventions. Such objective evidence is critical for demonstrating to our clients, health care payers, and others the benefits of occupational therapy.*

4.18.6 Bev — Session 3, Implementing Adaptive Occupation Related to the Clothes Rack and the Shoes

The following Monday, we telephoned the apartment manager who agreed with our plan. The manager preferred that an employee of the apartment building install the new clothes rack and remove the door of Bev's closet. The manager asked only that we mark Bev's closet so that they would know exactly where we wanted the rack. We also called her daughter to discuss with her both the clothes rack and the shoes. Her daughter willingly agreed to not only purchase the clothes

[29] The term *logit* refers to linear log-odds probability units (*log-it*). When an occupational therapist administers the AMPS, he or she enters the person's raw ordinal item scores for each ADL task performed into his or her personal copy of the AMPS computer-scoring software (Three Star Press, 2005). This software is then converts the person's raw scores to equal interval, linear measures of ADL ability — one measure for ADL motor ability and one measure for ADL process ability (Fisher, 2006a).

rack for her mother. She also mentioned that she had recently seen one at a local hardware store, and thought that it was not very expensive. She also agreed to meet with us to learn more about what needed to be done to Bev's shoes.

That afternoon, her daughter called, saying she had bought the rack. We called Bev and arranged to meet her and her daughter the next day (session 3). This enabled us to have Bev try reaching for clothing from the rack when we placed it a various heights, and then to mark the wall when we found the height that Bev preferred. As Bev was not feeling well, we did not take the time to have her take off or put on her shoes. We did, however, show her daughter that one of Bev's problems was reaching the Velcro® straps on her shoes. Her daughter told us that Bev used to have other shoes that were easier for her to put on, but that the physical therapist had the orthotist revise them as Bev now needed more support. Bev's daughter agreed to talk with the physical therapist or the orthotist about her mother's shoes.

4.18.7 Case Example: Bev — Session 4, Reevaluating for Enhanced Occupational Performance

That Friday, when we visited Bev for her fourth occupational therapy session, we began by sharing with Bev the results of our AMPS observation. She then shared with us that the new clothes rack already had been installed. Bev wanted to "see how it goes — do you think it will be better?" so we transitioned to observing Bev reach for and remove clothes from her newly installed clothes rack. With the door removed from her closet, she was able to move her wheelchair into the closet with minimal increase in physical effort and minimal inefficiency. Once positioned in front of her clothes, she began reaching for and removing one piece of clothing after another, saying "I have to put them where they belong. The man who put my clothes back in the rack put them all in the wrong places." Bev repositioned five garments efficiently and without increased physical effort or need to pause to rest.

If Bev, while reaching for and removing the clothes, had continued to demonstrate actions that she did not perform effectively, we would have redefined/described those actions that were ineffective and cycled back and reentered the OTIPM (see Figure 15). Since her performance was now effective and Bev had met her goal related to retrieving garments from her closet (see Documentation Example 5, Goal 3), we chose to exit the model in relation to ***that*** *goal. Instead, our plan was to reenter the model at the point of observing and implementing yet another performance analysis — one related to "taco lasagna"* *(see Figure 15). We also recognized that we would need to document the effectiveness of our intervention in our next progress note.*

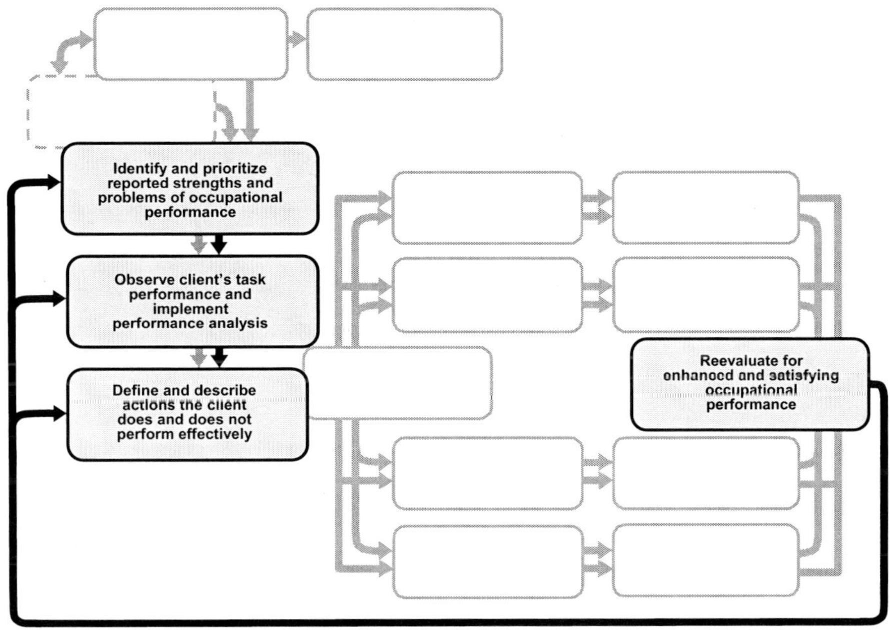

Figure 15. **Options for cycling back and reentering the occupational therapy intervention process.**

4.18.8 Case Example: Bev — Session 4, Evaluating and Implementing Intervention Related to Cooking

After we observed Bev reposition garments on her new clothes rack, she proceeded to prepare the taco lasagna. As we were not implementing a standardized performance analysis of her ability to cook, only an informal performance analysis of her ability to (a) stir and (b) remove hot pans from the oven, we had the opportunity to ***repeatedly enter the cycle*** *(i.e., have two "layers" of the OTIPM active simultaneously) and (a) define/describe actions Bev did not perform effectively, (b) define/clarify the cause, (c) select a model, (d) plan intervention, and (e) reevaluate for enhanced occupational performance (see Figures 12 and 15).*

For example, as Bev began to cut up the onion and green pepper for the lasagna, she used a small table 35 cm by 50 cm (13.5 inches by 19.5 inches). Already sitting on the table was a box of tissues, a package of ground meat, a paper plate, a can of beans, and a glass of water. The result was that her workspace was extremely crowded. Moreover, as she worked, she held her arms persistently abducted to 90 degrees at her shoulders. This resulted in her assuming awkward arm and body positions as she cut the vegetables. As we clarified the cause, we determined that the limited space on her kitchen counter seemed to contribute to her decision to use the small table. Although lower than her counters, the height of the table appeared to be the reason Bev held her arms in an awkward and inefficient position.

The students chose to intervene by selecting the compensatory model, and planning and implementing adaptive occupation, recommending to Bev that she use another small table that was in the living room. It was slightly larger, lighter in weight, and lower in height. Bev agreed to try cutting the vegetables on the second table. Our reevaluation revealed that her actions were now efficient, and Bev experienced only minimal difficulty.

Other examples of our reentering the cycle occurred when Bev was opening the can of beans and when she attempted to stir the taco mixture in the pan on the stove top. She again demonstrated difficulty positioning her body appropriately for the task and supporting task objects securely. The cause seemed to be the height of the work surfaces. With cueing from the students to try to again use the lower, lightweight table, Bev's problems were largely overcome.

Once we determined that the use of the lower, lighter table worked, Bev, the students, and I proceeded to address the issue of where Bev might store it. Together, we agreed to move a small cabinet in which Bev stored her medications into the living room, immediately to the right side of the refrigerator, and to store the small table in the vacant space left by the removed cabinet on the left side of the refrigerator. We also observed that Bev could place the table in its new storage position and remove it independently and efficiently, with minimal increased effort. In fact, Bev was able to lift the table and transport it to whatever location in the kitchen she preferred to have it as she continued to finish preparing the taco lasagna.

By the time Bev had finished making the taco lasagna, we had determined that while she was sitting in her wheelchair, she (a) was unable to safely bend forward, reach, support, and transport pans from the oven and required assistance; (b) was unable to independently adjust the dials on the oven or the burners of the stove top; (c) and was able to safely and efficiently stir food as long as she placed the pan on the small, lower table. Otherwise, Bev demonstrated moderate difficulty and inefficiency during the process of making taco lasagna before we implemented adaptive occupation and minimal difficulty and minimal inefficiency after we implemented adaptive occupation. Bev did not attempt to stand, so her earlier problems related to minimal safety risk when standing were not a factor.

At the end of our session, we talked with Bev about our recommendation that she not use the stove top or oven unless someone else was present. She expressed some dissatisfaction with the idea of not being able to cook hot meals independently. We discussed with her the possibility of cooking hot meals using her microwave oven and her electric frying pan, and we developed a plan to engage Bev in more meal preparation activities over the next few visits. This would enable us to (a) provide more opportunities for restorative and/or acquisitional occupation; (b) continue to implement adaptive occupation, when appropriate; (c) provide Bev with opportunities to practice and generalize newly learned skills and compensatory strategies; and (d) assess Bev's ability to prepare hot meals using the microwave oven and electric frying pan. Our summary progress note for our first four visits is shown in Documentation Example 10. Once again, we used "occupation first" language.

4.19 Reevaluate for Enhanced Occupational Performance

At regular intervals, after restorative, acquisitional, and/or adaptive occupation have been implemented, the client's occupational performance is reevaluated. During intervention, reevaluations most often focus on assessing whether or not a specific intervention was effective or a specific goal was met. They may, therefore, be more informal. At time of discharge, and when possible during intervention, it is important that we implement more formal, standardized reevaluations to document the effectiveness of occupational therapy interventions. Such reevaluations may include indices of client satisfaction, such as the COPM, but is it also critical that we again use performance analyses to verify whether or not the client has met his or her goals. If the performance analysis implemented during the reevaluation results in the identification of additional problems, the actions the person cannot perform effectively must be redefined/described and the cycle of defining/clarifying the cause, selecting a model, and so on, is repeated (see Figures 12 and 15).

Documentation Example 10: Bev: Summary Progress Report for First Four Visits

Summary Progress Report

S: "I could do that, but I haven't really tried it" (regarding cooking meals in microwave or electric skillet rather than in oven or on stove top).

O: Bev seen four times since start of care for therapeutic occupation to increase activity tolerance, collaborative consultation, education, adaptation, and AMPS assessment. Bev seen this date to address concerns related to hot meal preparation.

A: Bev is minimally unsafe and requires marked physical assistance when standing and attempting to stir foods. To prevent falls, she must use one hand to support herself when standing, and is therefore unable to stabilize the pan with one hand while stirring with the other. She is able to stir foods from a seated position (using a nonskid surface under the pan) independently, safely, and with minimal increase in effort. Bev requires marked physical assistance to remove, support, and transport hot foods from the oven, and is not safe to do so independently. Bev's progress to date is summarized below:

Goal	Baseline Status	Current Status
1. Don right shoe independently, efficiently, with minimal increase in physical effort, stopping to rest no more than 3 times	Moderately inefficient, moderate increase in physical effort, stopped to rest 5 times	Per baseline status; continue goal
2. Retrieve garments from closet independently, minimal increase in physical effort, stopping to rest no more than 1 time	Moderate increase in physical effort, from wheelchair with dressing stick; stopped to rest 3 times	Minimal increase in physical effort, no stops to rest; discontinue goal
3. Stand/retrieve objects in kitchen safely, with minimal increase in physical effort, stopping to rest no more than 1 time	Minimally unsafe when standing and moderate increase in physical effort; stopped to rest 2 times	Possible safety risk remains, minimal increase in physical effort, stops to rest 1-2 times, continue goal
4. Manage oxygen tubing efficiently, without it getting tangled in wheelchair	Minimally inefficient	Efficient with occasional verbal cue; discontinue goal
5. Stand/stir foods safely, independently, with only minimal increase in physical effort	Minimally unsafe, requires frequent physical assistance when standing to stir	Independent, safe, and only minimal increase in physical effort when seated to stir; continue goal
Remove/transport hot foods from oven safely (Bev's priority, not established as a goal	Unsafe, resulting in constant need for physical assistance	Unsafe, resulting in constant need for physical assistance

Documentation Example 10 (continued)

> *Bev is demonstrating good progress towards her goals and remains motivated to continue. She is not safe when removing or transporting hot foods from the oven, and should not attempt to do so without assistance. It may be beneficial for Bev to stir foods only when sitting.*
>
> ***P:*** *Recommend that Bev sit rather than stand when stirring foods. Assess Bev's ability to cook hot meals using microwave and electric frying pan. Continue goals 1 and 3; discontinue goals 2 and 4; add goal 5. Continue, as tolerated, per intervention plan, with emphasis on carryover of adaptive strategies into multiple tasks.*

If the client has met the goal, or the goal is discontinued, the occupational therapist can reenter the cycle by collaborating with the client to establish new priorities, and from there, progress to observing and implementing a performance analysis of the person performing the new task. Finally, documentation of the effectiveness of our occupational therapy interventions is a critical step toward communicating the unique role of occupational therapy as well as justifying payment of occupational therapy services by health care payers.

4.20 Discharge the Client

When the client's goals have been met, the client's progress plateaus, societal constraints prevent the continuation of occupational therapy services, or for any other reasons occupational therapy services do not seem warranted, the client is discharged. ***Since discharge may occur at any point in the occupational therapy intervention process*** (e.g., after establishing the client-centered performance context and determining the client has no need for occupational therapy services), ***discharge is not shown as a step in Chapter 1, Figure 5*** (see also the Appendix, Section 8.2, where discharge is included).

4.21 Case Example: Bev — Discharging the Client

Unfortunately, after our fourth visit, Bev was rehospitalized due to unspecified medical problems. As a result, we ceased our intervention with her and discharged her from occupational therapy. In our discharge summary, we recorded that she was discharged due to hospitalization and that her status toward her occupational therapy goals was per our summary progress note (see Documentation Example 10). We also recommended that she be referred to occupational therapy when her medical status stabilized.

4.22 Conclusions

In an environment of decreased health care monies, managed care, and shortened periods of rehabilitation, there are increased demands to implement cost-effective interventions. We must, therefore, make every effort to enable our clients to achieve maximum gains within the limited time available. While restorative occupation remains a vital aspect of occupational therapy, we must also recognize that the only way to achieve client goals in the limited time available is to introduce acquisitional and adaptive occupation and consultation from day one. ***Restoration is time consuming, and there is growing evidence that restoration may have limited effects on functional outcomes***.

We need to make a philosophical shift. We may need to let go of the type of thinking that is driven by a focus on restoration of underlying impairments and body function limitations. Instead, we need to focus on what the person wants and needs to do, and work with the person to enable him or her to perform tasks that are meaningful to the person and in a manner that brings satisfaction. This means that we need to rethink what is really important from the perspective of the person — occupational performance or his or her underlying limitations. We need to ***rethink the assessment process, using a true top–down approach that focuses on occupation***. We need to revise our intervention strategies and focus more on adaptation, education, and collaborative consultation and less on restoration. If we focus directly on occupational performance through acquisitional occupation and compensation, restoration may still occur as a secondary benefit. Moreover, just as in Bev's case, we can always stress acquisitional and adaptive occupation, but simultaneously implement restorative occupation.

When we do focus on restoration, we need to tie our interventions to our philosophical base through the application of restoration through engagement in occupation. The use of simulated occupation, whether in the form of simulative restorative, simulated acquisitional, or simulated adaptive occupation should only be used when engagement is naturalistic task performance is not possible. ***Preparation***

and rote practice/exercise lack sound foundations in our philosophical base; we must use them as infrequently as possible. Finally, we need to recognize the need to set goals and document efficacy in terms of occupational performance and not underlying person factors and body functions.

In this chapter, I have shown how a *true top–down process model*, one which simultaneously promotes both client-centered and occupation-based practice, can be used to guide the reasoning of occupational therapists as we provide services for our clients. Best practice in occupational therapy includes offering our clients services that are both of the highest possible quality and are cost effective. It is my belief that if occupational therapists use the OTIPM, they can achieve both. More specifically, our occupational therapy programs will be of higher quality when we provide services in a manner that is client-centered, and we use occupation-based assessments and interventions. Moreover, when we follow a true top–down evaluation process, we save time (and money) by avoiding the administration unneeded evaluations (especially evaluations focused on defining/clarifying the cause of the client's problems with occupational performance.

There is emerging evidence that evaluations and interventions implemented based on the OTIPM yield positive results in the form of enhanced occupational performance and goal attainment (Fisher, Atler, & Potts, 2007; Hällgren & Kottorp, 2005; Kottorp, Hällgren, Bernspång, & Fisher, 2003; Munkholm, 2008). To date, however, there is a lack of evidence that suggests that one process model is better than another. It is my hope, therefore, that future research will focus on enabling us to determine if our choice of process models yields different results.

5. OTIPM AS A REASONING MODEL FOR EVALUATING SOCIAL INTERACTION SKILLS — CASE EXAMPLE: BEN

by
Anne G. Fisher
Lou Ann Griswold

5.1 Chapter Overview

In the preceding chapter, I presented, in detail, the OTIPM as a model that can guide the occupational therapist's reasoning as he or she progresses through the various phases of ongoing occupational therapy services. The case example used in Chapter 4 was an older woman who had problems of occupational performance associated primarily with ADL motor and ADL process skills. In this chapter, I present yet another application of OTIPM, but with a focus on a man whose problems with occupational performance are primarily related to social interaction. While I will review some of the key features of each step of the OTIPM, in this chapter, I will emphasize the use of a standardized performance analysis, the *Evaluation of Social Interaction Skills* (ESI) (Fisher & Griswold, 2009), and the documentation thereof. As I will demonstrate, the reasoning process is the same as if the occupational therapist uses a nonstandardized performance analysis (see Chapter 4, Sections 4.10 to 4.12).

5.2 Implement Phase I of an Initial Occupational Therapy Evaluation

The ***first phase of an initial occupational therapy evaluation*** involves establishing the client-centered performance context in order to (a) identify the resources and limitations within the client's performance context; and (b) identify what occupational performances the client reports to be strengths and problems, and which ones the client wants to prioritize for further evaluation and potential intervention. The ***second phase*** involves implementing one or more performance analyses, and then defining and describing the actions of performance that were and were not effective. The ***final phase*** is to clarify or interpret the cause (see Chapter 1, Figure 5). To demonstrate how the occupational therapist uses the OTIPM to guide his or her professional reasoning in the process evaluating a client, and then documenting the results of a standardized performance analysis based on the ESI, I will use a case example based on a person named Ben.[30] He was referred by a community agency to his occupational therapist, Emma, because of concerns related to obtaining new employment. More specifically, the community agency sought Emma's input as to how they might best support Ben in finding a new job. The moment Emma learned this information, she initiated phase one of her evaluation, and started the process of establishing Ben's client-centered performance context.

When Emma met Ben and implemented an occupational therapy interview, she continued the process of establishing Ben's client-centered performance context. Her goal was to learn about Ben, the key resources and limitations in his performance context, and what types of task performances he reported were relevant and of concern. In this process, it became clear that Ben's problems with social interaction seemed to be a key factor not only in relation to seeking new employment, but also in relation to his more informal relationships with others, both at work and during leisure activities. Ben seemed to be quite aware of his problems, and felt that his problems at work and during leisure were related; he expressed concerns about both.

Emma, therefore, reasoned that implementing a performance analysis of Ben's social interaction skills as he engaged in relevant social exchanges would enable her to evaluate his quality of social interaction and better understand his problems. Thus, Emma suggested to Ben that she use the ESI to get a better idea of his problems when interacting with others. Ben agreed, and then collaborated with Emma as they determined what tasks that involve social interaction would be best for Emma to observe.

As Emma entered phase two of the occupational therapy evaluation, she began the process of implementing a performance analysis. She worked together with Ben and the community agency to arrange opportunities for Emma to observe Ben in natural settings. More specifically, the community agency had established relationships with a variety of companies who employ people with identified disabilities. Based on their recommendations, Emma arranged with one of these companies to interview Ben for a computer position. Both Ben and Mr. Rossi, the person who would do the interview, were aware that Emma would be in the room, and they arranged for her to sit to the side so as to be as unobtrusive as possible. It was critical that Emma's observation of Ben during the job interview provide her an opportunity to assess Ben's social interaction skills in the context of a real interview, without her disrupting the ongoing social interaction.

---

[30] This case example is adapted from Fisher & Griswold (2009), with permission.

To assess Ben's social interaction as he engaged in casual social conversations essential for full participation at work and during leisure activities with peers, Ben and Emma agreed that she observe Ben during a dinner with two of Ben's friends. One is a colleague from work and another (Grace) is a neighbor who lives nearby. Ben and his friends get together periodically, and eat dinner at a local restaurant that Ben especially likes as it is quiet. Emma and Ben arranged with Ben's friends to eat dinner together at this restaurant. They all agreed for Emma to sit at a nearby table while she unobtrusively observed them.

5.3 Document Phase I of the Initial Occupational Therapy Evaluation

Emma's documentation of phase one (i.e., the first four points shown in Chapter 3, Table 1) is shown in Documentation Example 11. During her interview with Ben, which lasted about 25 minutes, Emma gathered the information she needed to understand Ben and his concerns with occupational performance. The degree of detail to which this information will be documented will depend upon (a) how much information already exists in a person's record (e.g., there typically is no need to repeat information that is already documented), and (b) the type and format of documentation preferred by the occupational therapist and/or required by the work setting (e.g., narrative, computer-based data entry with fixed fields). Emma chose to use a narrative format. While she tried to keep her report relatively brief, she also wanted to include enough information so that those who read her report would be able to get a clear picture of Ben, his concerns, and why she evaluated his quality of social interaction in two different social contexts.

5.4 Summarize Ben's Overall (Global) Quality of Social Interaction

After the occupational therapist observes the person and implements a performance analysis (part of Phase II), he or she needs to ***document the client's baseline level of occupational performance — the person's quality performance, "doing," not what the person self-reports***. As discussed in Chapter 3, documentation of a person's baseline level of performance is critical for evidence-based practice, as each baseline statement provides a point-of-reference for both establishing realistic goals, and then determining whether the person met his or her goals, made progress toward his or her goals, or exceeded his or her goals. Again, the person's baseline quality of social interaction can be documented as one or more global baseline statements and/or as a

Documentation Example 11: Ben's ESI Evaluation Report — Reason for Referral, Relevant History, Reported Strengths and Problems with Occupational Performance, and Task Performances Prioritized for Further Evaluation

OCCUPATIONAL THERAPY EVALUATION

Name: Ben Sample
Date of evaluation: March 4, 2008
Occupational therapist: Emma Andersen

Reason for Referral

Ben was referred to occupational therapy by a community agency that provides supports and services to adults with disabilities. Ben sought their help in seeking new employment where he can use his computer skills. The community agency requested an occupational therapy evaluation and recommendations related to how to support Ben in obtaining new employment.

Relevant History

Ben is 23 years of age and has Asperger's syndrome. He has a university degree in computer science. He reports that he excelled in his coursework, but "struggled with getting along with other students." Ben currently lives alone in his own apartment, and works full time as a delivery person for a local florist, but is dissatisfied with his job as it is not related to his interests or prior training in computer science. He enjoys golf, but rarely plays. He reports that he spends most of his leisure time alone, going for walks by himself and playing computer games online, because of difficulty "fitting in" with his peers. He would prefer to play golf with others his own age, but is never invited to play. He occasionally socializes with a co-worker from work and a neighbor, whom he refers to as his "not so close" friends. Otherwise, he reports that interacting with others at work is a problem. He also has an older brother whom Ben reports meeting about once a month. Unlike with his friends and coworkers, Ben reports that he has a good relationship and social interactions with his brother. Ben appears to have a clear sense of his strengths and limitations as well as his desires for his immediate future.

Reported Strengths and Problems with Daily Life Task Performance

Ben reports that his strengths include performing tasks that involve the use of his math and computer skills. He is able to perform all personal care and household tasks independently, as he has no need to interact with others. In contrast, Ben reports problems related to tasks that involve social interaction. He says that he went for two interviews with large computer companies but "did not do well in the interview process." He also reports problems when socializing with his friends during leisure activities, and during informal social interactions at work.

Activities Prioritized for Further Evaluation

Ben identified two tasks that involve social interaction as priorities for further evaluation: (a) interacting with someone in the context of being interviewed for a job, and (b) engaging in casual conversation while eating a meal together with friends or during coffee breaks at work. The *Evaluation of Social Interaction* was used to assess Ben's quality of social interaction.

series of more detailed specific baseline statements. In this section, I will discuss documenting the global baseline. I will discuss documenting the specific baseline in more detail below.

To document a global baseline, the occupational therapist can use the nonstandardized scoring criteria included in Chapter 6, Section 6.5 (for social interaction, see especially Section 6.5.5). When the occupational therapist uses the ESI, he or she records similar summary information on Page 1 of the ESI Score Form for each social interaction observed (see Documentation Examples 12 and 13). If the person's overall quality of social interaction was similar during both social interactions, the occupational therapist may choose to combine them into a single global summary baseline statement.

For example, Emma could have documented Ben's global baseline as follows:

When Ben was observed during a job interview with an unfamiliar social partner, as well as when interacting socially with friends while eating dinner together, Ben demonstrated markedly inappropriate social interaction that resulted in a very uncomfortable atmosphere that was detrimental to the ongoing social interactions.

5.5 Define and Describe the Social Interaction Items Ben Does and Does Not Perform Effectively

Sometimes, documenting a person's global baseline level of performance is sufficient. In most instances, however, it is desirable or necessary to further clarify the person's global baseline by documenting a more specific baseline level of performance. More importantly, as I will discuss below, documenting a more detailed specific baseline can help to guide the collaborative process of setting client-centered goals and planning occupation-based interventions. ***The specific baseline is based upon determining which social interaction skills were effective and which were most ineffective***. This information comes from our standardized or nonstandardized ratings for each of the social interaction items included in Chapter 6, Section 6.4. When the occupational therapist uses the ESI, there are detailed scoring criteria that guide the determination of the raw scores given to each ESI item (see Documentation Examples 12 and 13). More specifically, just as we did with Bev (see Chapter 4, Section 4.12.3), during this phase, the occupational therapist (a) uses his or her professional reasoning skills to reflect on what he or she observed during each naturalistic social exchange, and (b) identifies the items that most reflect the person's problem areas.

Documentation Example 12: Ben's ESI Score Form for Social Interaction 1 — *Sharing Information*

EVALUATION OF SOCIAL INTERACTION SCORE FORM (Page 1)

Name: Ben

therapist: Emma

Gender: X Male ____Female

Date of evaluation: March 4, 2008

Date of birth: May 16, 1984 **Age:** 23

diagnosis: Asperger's

Secondary diagnosis: ____________

Observation number: X 1 ____2 ____3 ____4

Intended purpose of social interaction:
- ____ Gathering information (GI)
- X Sharing information (SI)
- ____ Problem solving/Decision making (PD)
- ____ Collaborating/Producing (CP)
- ____ Acquiring goods and services (AG)
- ____ Conversing socially/Small talk (CS)

Social interaction code: SI-4

Detailed task description: Interviewing for a job at supported employment

Time of day:
____ Morning X Afternoon ____ Evening

Familiarity of the physical environment:
- ____ Familiar
- ____ Somewhat familiar
- X Unfamiliar

Degree of expected structure:
- ____ High structure
- X Relaxed structure
- ____ "Free" structure

Noise level:
- X Quiet
- ____ Moderate noise
- ____ Extreme noise

Number of social partners: 1

Primary social partner: Mr. Rossi

Familiarity of primary the social partner:
- ____ Familiar
- ____ Somewhat familiar
- X Unknown/not familiar

of primary the social partner:
- X *Expert/supervisor/teacher/service provider*
- ____ Receiver of services/customer
- ____ Friend/colleague/classmate
- ____ Family member/relative
- ____ Other acquaintance

Age of primary social partner:
- ____ Child (10 years and under)
- ____ Adolescent (11 to 17 years)
- X Adult (18 to 64 years)
- ____ Older adult (65 years and above)

Social partner's overall quality of social interaction:
- X Appropriate
- ____ Questionable
- ____ Minimally inappropriate
- ____ Moderately inappropriate
- ____ Markedly inappropriate

Overall comfort level of the social interaction
- ____ Generally comfortable
- ____ Questionable if comfortable
- ____ Uncomfortable
- X Very uncomfortable

Person's overall quality of social interaction
- ____ Appropriate
- ____ Questionable
- ____ Minimally inappropriate
- ____ Moderately inappropriate
- X Markedly inappropriate

Documentation Example 12 (continued)

EVALUATION OF SOCIAL INTERACTION SCORE FORM (Page 2)

ITEM RAW SCORES

Initiating and Terminating Social Interaction	Score (circled)	Comment
1. Approaches/Starts	4 3 (2) 1	pauses before responding
2. Concludes/Disengages	4 3 (2) 1	ends somehat abruptly
Producing Social Interaction		
3. Produces Speech	(4) 3 2 1	
4. Gesticulates	4 3 2 (1)	no gestures
5. Speaks Fluently	4 3 (2) 1	fast, uneven tempo
Physically Supporting Social Interaction		
6. Turns Toward	4 3 (2) 1	turns body, not face
7. Looks	4 3 2 (1)	no eye contact
8. Places Self	(4) 3 2 1	
9. Touches	4 3 (2) 1	delay to shake hands
10. Regulates	4 3 (2) 1	repetitive hand movements
Shaping Content of Social Interaction		
11. Questions	(4) 3 2 1	
12. Replies	4 3 (2) 1	too little detail
13. Discloses	(4) 3 2 1	
14. Expresses Emotion	4 3 2 (1)	no emotion
15. Disagrees	(4) 3 2 1	
16. Thanks	4 3 2 (1)	does not thank

Maintaining Flow of Social Interaction	Score (circled)	Comment
17. Transitions	(4) 3 2 1	
18. Times Response	(4) 3 2 1	
19. Times Duration	4 3 2 (1)	too brief, partner asks for clarification
20. Takes Turns	(4) 3 2 1	
Verbally Supporting Social Interaction		
21. Matches Language	(4) 3 2 1	
22. Clarifies	(4) 3 2 1	
23. Acknowledges/ Encourages	4 3 (2) 1	does not encourage
24. Empathizes	(4) 3 2 1	
Adapting Social Interaction		
25. Heeds	(4) 3 2 1	
26. Accommodates	4 3 2 (1)	does not prevent problems
27. Benefits	4 3 2 (1)	problems persist

Additional comments:

Documentation Example 13: Ben's ESI Score Form for Social Interaction 2 — *Conversing socially/ Small talk*

EVALUATION OF SOCIAL INTERACTION SCORE FORM (Page 1)

Name: Ben

therapist: Emma

Gender: X Male ____Female

Date of evaluation: March 4, 2008

Date of birth: May 16, 1984 **Age:** 23

diagnosis: Asperger's

Secondary diagnosis: ____________

Observation number: ____1 X 2 ____3 ____4

Intended purpose of social interaction:
- ____ Gathering information (GI)
- ____ Sharing information (SI)
- ____ Problem solving/Decision making (PD)
- ____ Collaborating/Producing (CP)
- ____ Acquiring goods and services (AG)
- X Conversing socially/Small talk (CS)

Social interaction code: CS-1

Detailed task description: Eating dinner with friend and colleague

Time of day:
____ Morning ____ Afternoon X Evening

Familiarity of the physical environment:
- X Familiar
- ____ Somewhat familiar
- ____ Unfamiliar

Degree of expected structure:
- ____ High structure
- ____ Relaxed structure
- X "Free" structure

Noise level:
- X Quiet
- ____ Moderate noise
- ____ Extreme noise

Number of social partners: 2

Primary social partner: Grace

of primary the social partner:
- X Familiar
- ____ Somewhat familiar
- ____ Unknown/not familiar

Status of primary the social partner:
- ____ *Expert/supervisor/teacher/service provider*
- ____ Receiver of services/customer
- X Friend/colleague/classmate
- ____ Family member/relative
- ____ Other acquaintance

Age of primary social partner:
- ____ Child (10 years and under)
- ____ Adolescent (11 to 17 years)
- X Adult (18 to 64 years)
- ____ Older adult (65 years and above)

Social partner's overall quality of social interaction:
- ____ Appropriate
- ____ Questionable
- ____ Minimally inappropriate
- ____ Moderately inappropriate
- X Markedly inappropriate

Overall comfort level of the social interaction
- ____ Generally comfortable
- ____ Questionable if comfortable
- ____ Uncomfortable
- X Very uncomfortable

Person's overall quality of social interaction
- ____ Appropriate
- ____ Questionable
- ____ Minimally inappropriate
- ____ Moderately inappropriate
- X Markedly inappropriate

Documentation Example 13 (continued)

EVALUATION OF SOCIAL INTERACTION SCORE FORM (Page 2)

ITEM RAW SCORES

Item	Score (circled)	Comment
Initiating and Terminating Social Interaction		
1. Approaches/Starts	4	
2. Concludes/Disengages	4 3 2 1 (none circled)	N/A
Producing Social Interaction		
3. Produces Speech	4	
4. Gesticulates	1	exaggerated gestures
5. Speaks Fluently	2	uneven tempo
Physically Supporting Social Interaction		
6. Turns Toward	2	turns body, not face
7. Looks	2	looks down, away
8. Places Self	4	
9. Touches	4	
10. Regulates	2	repetitive hand movements
Shaping Content of Social Interaction		
11. Questions	4	
12. Replies	1	does not reply to partner
13. Discloses	4	
14. Expresses Emotion	1	no emotion, then too much
15. Disagrees	1	disagrees with inapprop anger
16. Thanks	4	

Item	Score (circled)	Comment
Maintaining Flow of Social Interaction		
17. Transitions	1	transitions to markedly irrelevant
18. Times Response	2	interrupts partner
19. Times Duration	2	messages too short
20. Takes Turns	1	does not take turn, partner dominates
Verbally Supporting Social Interaction		
21. Matches Language	4	
22. Clarifies	4	
23. Acknowledges/ Encourages	2	sometimes does not nod, smile
24. Empathizes	1	no messages to support partner
Adapting Social Interaction		
25. Heeds	1	transitions to markedly irrelevant
26. Accommodates	1	does not prevent problems
27. Benefits	1	problems persist

Additional comments:

To identify items that best reflect the person's problem areas, the occupational therapist typically begins by making a list of all social interaction skills (i.e., ESI items) that were scored as ineffective (ESI score = 2) or severely limited (ESI score = 1) in one or more of the observations, and then prioritizes up to 10 social interaction skills that most reflect the person's diminished quality of social interaction.

For example, Emma reviewed Ben's raw scores, and made a list of those ESI items that were ineffective or severely limited. Emma then used her professional reasoning to identify those items that she felt were most impacting his quality of performance. These skills she marked with a check mark (√) (see Table 9).

Notice that when Emma identified the items that most impacted Ben's quality of social interaction, she did not just chose those that she had scored = 1. Instead, Emma considered Ben's performance during each social interaction in relation to the intended purpose, his social partners, and the setting. She then chose those that she felt best captured his problems with social interaction. In some cases, she considered items she had scored = 2 to be more clinically meaningful than were ones she had scored = 1 (e.g., Thanks, Transitions). For example, while she had scored Thanks = 1 for the job interview, Ben demonstrated no problem with Thanks during his dinner conversation. Moreover, Emma felt that Ben's failure to thank Mr. Rossi at the end of the job interview did not best reflect Ben's key problem areas.

During this phase of the professional reasoning process, the occupational therapist will also want to make note of the social interaction skills that are relative strengths. When evaluating for relative strengths, it can also be informative to compare performance between different social contexts (e.g., familiar vs. unfamiliar partner or environment, quality of social interaction of the primary social partner).

For example, Emma noted that Ben had received scores = 4 on Produces Speech, Places Self, Questions, Discloses, Matches Language, and Clarifies for both social exchanges. She also noted that Ben's overall quality of performance was somewhat better when he was engaged in the job interview with Mr. Rossi, a social partner with good social interaction skills. The skills that Emma judged to be most supported by Mr. Rossi's quality of social interaction were Disagrees, Transitions, Times Response, Takes Turns, and Heeds.

Emma was aware that she could also have viewed the differences in Ben's quality of social interaction from the standpoint of the negative impact of Grace's markedly inappropriate quality of social interaction. She reasoned, however, that

(a) she already had identified several skills that are problems for Ben, and (b) by presenting these differences from a positive perspective, she could provide better evidence to support Ben's potential to benefit from occupational therapy intervention.

Table 9 Ben's Social Interaction Skills that were Ineffective (I) or Severely Limited (SL)

Sharing information: job interview		Conversing socially/Small talk: eating dinner with friends	
Approaches/Starts (I)		Gesticulates (SL)	√
Concludes/Disengages (I)		Speaks Fluently (I)	
Gesticulates (SL)	√	Turns Toward (I)	
Speaks Fluently (I)		Looks (I)	√
Turns Toward (I)	√	Regulates (I)	√
Looks (SL)	√	Replies (SL)	√
Touches (I)		Expresses Emotion (SL)	√
Regulates (I)	√	Disagrees (SL)	√
Replies (I)	√	Transitions (SL)	
Expresses Emotion (SL)	√	Times Response (I)	
Thanks (SL)		Times Duration (I)	√
Times Duration (SL)	√	Takes Turns (SL)	√
Acknowledges/Encourages (I)		Acknowledges/Encourages (SL)	
Accommodates (SL)	√	Heeds (I)	
Benefits (SL)	√	Accommodates (SL)	√
		Benefits (SL)	√

5.6 Summarize Ben's Specific Baseline Quality of Social Interaction

After the occupational therapist has identified up to 10 social interaction items that best reflect the person's diminished quality of social interaction, the next step is to ***group those skills into three to five clusters of items that reflect interrelated behaviors***. The occupational therapist then writes a short statement summarizing the key problem reflected by each cluster. ***Those cluster summary statements become the basis for documenting the person's specific baseline quality of social interaction. It is critical,***

therefore, that the cluster summary statements be written in a form that describe observable behavior.

For example, Emma created the following cluster summary statements:

- ***Cluster 1– Turns Toward** and **Looks**: Ben turned his body but not his face toward his social partners, and did not make any eye contact with his social partners throughout his job interview and his dinner conversation.*
- ***Cluster 2 – Replies, Times Duration**, and **Takes Turns**: Ben frequently responded to his social partners with only one to two word messages that lacked needed information or detail, and on two occasions during his dinner conversation, he sent no reply to his social partner's messages. As a result, Ben allowed his social partners to dominate the social interaction during the dinner conversation.*
- ***Cluster 3 – Regulates** and **Gesticulates**: Throughout both social exchanges, Ben demonstrated constant repetitive hand movements. As a result, he did not use his hands to make gestures to support the information he communicated during his job interview. When engaged in conversation with his friends during dinner, he either made no gestures at all, or on two occasions, he had such exaggerated gestures that they were markedly disruptive to the ongoing social interaction.*
- ***Cluster 4 – Expresses Emotion** and **Disagrees**: Throughout his job interview and during the majority of the dinner conversation, Ben expressed no emotion. On one occasion, during the dinner conversation, he exploded with anger and yelled when he disagreed with one of his social partners.*
- ***Cluster 5 – Accommodates** and **Benefits**: Ben did not anticipate or prevent his problems with social interaction from occurring, and many of his problems persisted throughout the social interactions.*

When documenting the person's baseline quality of performance, the occupational therapist needs to also consider the benefits of creating cluster statements that summarize the person's strengths of social interaction.

For example, Emma felt that there were three additional key clusters that reflected Ben's strengths during social interaction, which she summarized as follows:

- ***Cluster 1 – Produces Speech** and **Matches Language**: Throughout both social exchanges, Ben spoke clearly and used language appropriate to his social partners and the social context.*
- ***Cluster 2 – Times Response** and **Takes Turns**: When he interacted with a socially competent partner during a more structured social exchange, a job interview, Ben took his turn in a timely and appropriate manner, without interrupting his social partner.*
- ***Cluster 3 – Transitions** and **Heeds**: During the more structured job interview, Ben kept the content of his messages focused on the intended purpose of the social interaction, and the topic being discussed, without transitioning to an irrelevant or inappropriate topic.*

The specific baseline summary statements Emma wrote are observable. Therefore, in most work settings, they would also be considered to be measurable. In other settings, Emma may need to add even more detail for her baseline summary statements to be considered measurable. Some examples of more detailed, observable, and measurable baseline summary statements include the following:

- During a 15 minute job interview and a 20 minute informal dinner conversation with two friends, Ben continuously turned his body toward his social partners, but did not make any eye contact throughout both social interactions.
- During a 15 minute job interview and a 20 minute informal dinner conversation with two friends, Ben responded to 75% of his social partner's questions and comments with only one to two word messages that lacked needed information or detail, and on two occasions he sent no reply to his social partner's messages.

Whatever the specific demands of the occupational therapist's work setting, it remains ***imperative that the documented baseline is observable and measurable***. Emma's documentation of Ben's baseline quality of social interaction is shown in Documentation Example 14. To write her baseline, she merely linked together her global baseline statement and her first five cluster summary statements that described his specific baseline. She then ended by linking in her three cluster statements that described some of Ben's strengths as support for her justification of Ben's potential to benefit from occupational therapy intervention.

Documentation Example 14: Ben's ESI Evaluation Report — Baseline Level of Social Interaction Skill and Recommendations for Occupational Therapy Intervention

OCCUPATIONAL THERAPY EVALUATION

(continued)

Name: Ben Sample

Results of the Evaluation of Social Interaction

When Ben was observed during a 15 minute job interview with an unfamiliar social partner, as well as during a 20 minute conversation with friends while eating dinner together, Ben demonstrated markedly inappropriate quality of social interaction that resulted in an uncomfortable atmosphere that was detrimental to the ongoing social exchanges. More specifically, Ben turned his body but not his face toward his social partners, and did not make any eye contact with his social partners throughout his job interview and his dinner conversation. Ben frequently responded to his social partners with only one or two word messages that lacked needed information or detail, and on two occasions during the dinner conversation he sent no reply to his social partner's messages. As a result, Ben allowed his friends to dominate the social interaction during the dinner conversation. Throughout both social exchanges, Ben demonstrated constant repetitive hand movements. As a result, he did not use his hands to make gestures to support the information he communicated during his job interview. When engaged in conversation with his friends during dinner, he either made no gestures at all, or on two occasions, he had such exaggerated gestures that they were markedly disruptive to the ongoing social interaction. Throughout his job interview and during the majority of the dinner conversation, Ben expressed no emotion. On one occasion, during the dinner conversation, he exploded with anger and yelled when he disagreed with one of his social partners. Finally, Ben did not anticipate and prevent his problems with social interaction from occurring, and many of his problems persisted throughout both social exchanges.

It is important to note that Ben also demonstrated a number of strengths during his social exchanges. For example, during both social exchanges, Ben spoke clearly and used language appropriate to his social partners and the type of social exchange. When he interacted with a socially competent partner during a more structured social exchange, the job interview, Ben took his turn in a timely and appropriate manner, without interrupting his social partner. He also kept the content of his messages focused on the intended purpose of the social interaction, and the topic being discussed, without transitioning to an irrelevant or inappropriate topic.

Recommendations

Ben appears to have good potential to benefit from occupational therapy intervention. His high level of motivation and apparent understanding of his strengths and problems with social interaction suggest that Ben has very good potential to build on his relative strengths to develop enhanced quality of social interaction for needed social interactions at work and during casual social interactions with friends and colleagues.

5.7 Develop Client-centered Goals Based on the Results of an ESI Observation

If the occupational therapist has recommended further services, he or she will need to begin the collaborative process of developing ***client-centered goals – the client's desired outcomes from occupational therapy interventions***. Goals must be client-centered. This means that the person, and when indicated, others in the client constellation, must be the ones who determine the goals. Goals must also be observable, measureable, and achievable. Most clients, however, lack the needed skills and/or find it hard to express clearly what it is they hope to achieve in a manner that is observable, measureable, and/or achievable. As a result, it is typically the occupational therapist who writes the goals. The occupational therapist may even suggest possible goals, building on his or her understanding of the client and the client's expressed desires. When he or she does suggest goals, the occupational therapist must also verify that the client agrees with the occupational therapist's suggestions before documenting them.

As we noted earlier, the occupational therapist's documentation of ***a person's baseline quality of social interaction*** included in the ESI evaluation report (see Documentation Example 14) ***provides a reference point to suggest observable and measurable goal statements***. That is, we believe that when the occupational therapist shares with the client the results of the ESI observations using observable, measurable descriptions of what he or she observed, these descriptions (i.e., each cluster summary statement and/or the global baseline statement) can each become the basis for a goal.

Obviously, the baseline statements need to be linked in a meaningful way to the client's expressed hopes and desires for the future.

For example, Emma was aware that Ben wanted to find a new job were he could use his computer skills, and "fit in" with his peers and "do more" with them. Emma also was aware that while these "goals" might well provide the context for Ben's goals, they were not yet expressed as observable, measureable, and achievable goals.

When Emma met with Ben and shared with him the results of the ESI, she also discussed how some of the behaviors she observed likely are contributing to the difficulties he has been having when applying for jobs and socializing with his peers. She engaged Ben in a discussion where they, together, considered the documented description of Ben's baseline quality of social interaction performance (see Documentation Example 14), and then identified which skills might best reflect the changes Ben hoped to achieve in order to improve his overall level of social interaction.

The next step was for Emma and Ben to write his goals together. Ben's input was especially important when determining the focus and content of his goals. Emma's role was to ensure that his goals were realistic and written in a form that was observable and measurable. More specifically, Ben and Emma began by considering the baseline observations that Emma included in her evaluation report. She and Ben then considered (a) which of these baseline behaviors was most important for Ben, and (b) what level of performance he hoped to achieve and Emma felt was possible.

While Ben was referred to Emma by the community agency in order to determine how to support Ben in finding the type of employment he was seeking, Ben and Emma felt that focusing on his social interactions with peers in more informal social contexts actually were more challenging for him, overall, than was the job interview. Ben's initial goals, therefore, focused on informal conversation. Ben felt, and Emma agreed, that if he could "practice" his skills with his friends, any improvements would likely carry over to his work environment. Emma, therefore, contacted the community agency to ensure that they agreed with this plan. The goals that Ben and Emma developed are shown in Documentation Example 15.

5.8 Develop Occupation-based Interventions

Once the client's goals are developed, the occupational therapist begins collaborating with the client to develop a plan for occupational therapy intervention that will enable the client to meet the goals that have been established. When reasoning about possibilities for interventions for Ben, Emma recommended that they begin with social skills training (acquisitional occupation) (see Chapter 2, Figure 8). Some of Ben's strengths seemed to be his motivation and his reasonably good insight. Emma reasoned, therefore, that restorative occupation (i.e., occupation-based interventions focused on his developing these underlying person factors and body functions) was not needed. Emma was also aware, if she found that Ben, in fact, did need to further develop these underlying capacitates, that Emma could also combine social skills training with strategies to, for example, enhance Ben's insight and awareness of his inappropriate behaviors. Finally, Emma reasoned that she likely would want to work with the community agency and any potential employer in the process of developing accommodations in the social environment within Ben's workplace (adaptive occupation), either where he is now working, or in any new workplace where he might obtain a new job (see Chapter 2, Figure 9).

Documentation Example 15: Ben's Goal Statements Based on the Results of the ESI

OCCUPATIONAL THERAPY EVALUATION
(continued)

Name: Ben Sample

Goals

During a 20 minute or greater informal social interaction (e.g., casual conversation with one to two work colleagues during a coffee break, dinner conversation with one or two friends), Ben will

- Make socially appropriate eye contact with his social partner at least 50% of the time
- Respond consistently to his social partners' comments and questions
- Make comments or answer questions with adequate information/detail at least 50% of the time
- Demonstrate repetitive hand gestures less than 25% of the time
- Use meaningful gestures to support his verbal message and not use exaggerated gestures that disrupt the social exchange
- Express disagreement with his social partner in a socially appropriate manner, without explosive anger or yelling

6. MOTOR, PROCESS, AND SOCIAL INTERACTION SKILLS

In this chapter, I present taxonomies of ***goal-directed actions*** (performance skills) that can be observed in most occupational performances. That is, the performance skills included in the OTIPM are divided into three taxonomies: ***motor skills***, ***process skills***, and ***social interaction skills***. As I define them, they are observable and goal-directed actions, the ***smallest observable units of occupational performance*** that are linked together one by one as we construct or compile a task performance. That is, if we think of a task performance as a chain of actions, then each observable performance skill becomes a link in that chain of actions — the task performance (see Figure 16).

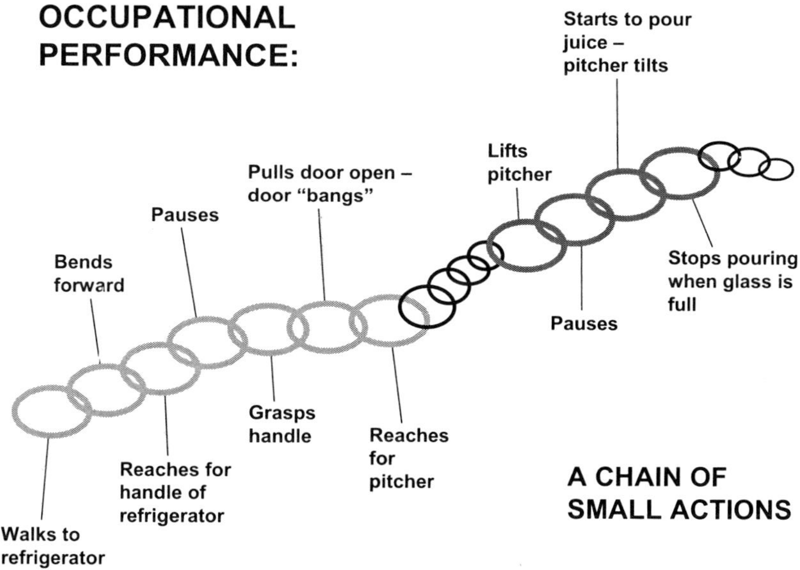

Figure 16. **Performance skills: Smallest observable units of occupational performance — links in a chain of actions performed one-by-one as the person "constructs" the overall task performance.**

This means that a task performance unfolds over time as each action is performed, one-by-one, one after another. That is, when we perform tasks, we perform a series of smaller, but observable actions over the course of the task performance. Said in slightly different words, each action is observable as part of the task performance, never as the underlying capacity needed to perform the action.[31] For example, to get ourselves a drink of juice, we must ***walk*** to the refrigerator, ***bend*** forward and ***reach*** out, grasp (***grip***) the handle of the refrigerator, and pull it open (***move***), pulling hard enough to get the door open, but not so hard as to have it "fling" open (***calibrate***). We then ***reach*** in, ***grip*** the pitcher of juice, ***lift*** it, and take it out of the refrigerator. We may then carry ***(transport)*** it to the counter and set it down without undue force (***calibrate***). And, as we

[31] This point may need further clarification because, with the publication of the second edition of the Framework (AOTA, 2008), motor, process, and social interaction performance skills were replaced with (a) motor and praxis skills, (b) sensory-perceptual skills, (c) emotional regulation skills, (d) cognitive skills, and (e) communication and social skills. The result was that the new Framework has reverted back to including both underlying capacities (body functions) and units of occupation under the construct "performance skills." Yet, *performance skills* pertain to the smallest observable units of occupation, *never* body functions (Fisher, 1998, 2006a, 2006b; Fisher & Griswold, 2009; Fisher & Kielhofner, 1995).

If I use *praxis* as an example, perhaps the difference between the smallest observable units of occupational performance and underlying body functions will become clear. Developmental dyspraxia is a disorder of planning and executing planned actions, especially "affecting the initiation, organization and performance of action" (Wikipedia, 2009). Within ICF (WHO, 2001), planning and carrying out plans (**b164**), and sequencing complex movements (**b176**) are mental functions. Only when we progress to the point of considering the performance of a task (e.g., writing a letter, making one's bed) do we progress to the level of observable activity and participation within ICF (for example, see **d210**, Undertaking a single task in ICF) (see also the Appendix, Table 10).

To evaluate for the presence of dyspraxia, we might ask a child to catch a ball with two hands or to hop in a series of circles placed on the floor. We cannot observe "planning," nor can we observe "executing" or "sequencing" per se. We can, however, observe "catching a ball" and "hoping in circles." Moreover, if the child has dyspraxia, we often observe that there is a delay before the child closes his or her hands on the ball to "catch it," resulting the ball not being caught or the ball hitting the child's chest. When that same child attempts to hop in the series of circles, we often observe that the child hesitates before initiating hopping, pauses before hopping into the next circle, begins to hop faster and faster, and starts to hop on the circles rather than hop with his or her foot within the circles. This is what we observe — delayed catching actions, not catching the ball, delays initiating hopping actions, discontinuous hopping actions, uneven speed of hopping actions, incorrect foot placement actions. Each of these actions can be considered to be a performance error, an action of performance that is "out of form" (Fisher, 1998). When we consider these observations as we attempt to interpret the cause (see Chapter 1, Figure 5), we might conclude that the child has dyspraxia. Our interpretation (dyspraxia) is not what we observed, it is our conclusion. If the child was very young, we might have interpreted what we observed in a very different manner — this child demonstrates age-appropriate praxis.

The very fact that we can have more than one interpretation of the same observations should be a signal to all of us that there is a clear distinction between what we observe and our interpretation. Now I add one more layer to our reasoning. Asking a child to catch a ball or hop in a series of circles on the floor is *not* occupation — the child was not engaged in the naturalistic performance of a chosen daily life task (e.g., playing basketball, playing hopscotch). This child was being evaluated by an occupational therapist and performed these actions because he or she was asked to. To evaluate performance skills, we must always evaluate the quality of the person's actions within the context of engagement is meaningful and/or purposeful activity. But this latter is not my key point. My key point pertains to an unfortunate source of confusion that has manifested itself in the new Framework.

carry out each of these small units of doing and interact with the environment and task objects, we must remain stable (***stabilize***) and not stumble or fall. Each of the words in bold italic is an example of an observable motor skill.

In a similar manner, we also can observe process skills. For example, continuing with our getting that drink from the refrigerator, an effective process requires that we ***initiate*** each action without pause (e.g., initiate walking over to the refrigerator, initiate reaching for the refrigerator door). Once we start an action, efficient performance requires that we ***continue*** that action through to completion without unnecessary pauses. For example, we continue reaching until we grasp the door; we continue carrying the juice to the counter until we are at the counter. We must also ***terminate*** our actions at the correct time, without premature stopping or going on too long. For example, we terminate pouring the juice once the glass is reasonably full and before juice spills over the rim. Finally, we ***sequence*** our actions in a logical order, opening the top of the pitcher before we pour the juice, not after. We also get a glass before we begin to pour the juice. We need to ***choose*** a glass and the pitcher of juice, ***gather*** them to the counter and ***organize*** that workplace so that the objects are not too close together or too far apart for effective performance. Before we even chose, we need to ***search*** for and ***locate*** the juice in the refrigerator and the glass in the cupboard. We ***heed*** when we carry out the "correct" task, doing what we said we would do, and doing it in a manner that is not out of form.

Finally, we carry out observable social interactions when we ***approach*** a social partner and ***start*** a conversation. As we engage in our social interaction, we ***turn toward*** and ***look*** at our partner. As we communicate, we ***produce speech*** and ***gesticulate*** (e.g., shake our heads, smile). We ***speak fluently***, ***take turns*** with our social partner, and speak for reasonable time periods (***times duration***), without "talking over" our social partner (***times response***), and so on.

The motor and process skills are derived from the Assessment of Motor and Process Skills (AMPS) (Fisher, 2006c) and the School Version of the Assessment of Motor and Process Skills (School AMPS) (Fisher et al., 2007). The evolution of the motor and process skills and their definitions began as a collaborative effort that occurred between 1987 and 1988 between Gary Kielhofner and myself. The first complete set of operational definitions of the motor and process skills were reported in 1989, in the first research edition of the AMPS (Fisher, 1989). Since that time, they have been incorporated into the Model of Human Occupation (Fisher & Kielhofner, 1995; Kielhofner, 2002, 2008), the OTIPM, and the original version of the Occupational Therapy Practice Framework (Framework) (AOTA, 2002). The definitions in the

Framework come from an earlier edition of the AMPS (Fisher, 2003). In the OTIPM, I have modified the definitions of the motor and process skills so that they can be used for informal evaluation of performance skills.

The development of the social interaction skills can be considered to have begun with the work of Doble and Magill-Evans (1992). During the next phase, building on the work of Doble and Magill-Evans, beginning in 1992, Englund (1997; Englund, Bernspång, & Fisher, 1995) developed the Assessment of Social Interaction (ASI) which included the first operational definitions for 25 social interaction skills. As with the motor and process skills, Englund's taxonomy of social interaction skills (as well as a taxonomy of communication and interaction skills) were incorporated into the Model of Human Occupation (Fisher & Kielhofner, 1995). In 2002, I began a process of refining and further clarifying the ASI items for inclusion in the OTIPM (Fisher, 2002/2006). As part of that process, I reviewed the actions listed in (a) the Communication and (b) the Interpersonal Interactions and Relationships domains of the International Classification of Functioning, Disability, and Health (ICF) (WHO, 2001). This resulted in several new items being added, and in others being revised. The resulting 27 items provided the basis for the new Evaluation of Social Interaction (ESI) (Fisher & Griswold, 2009), and these new social interaction skills are included in this version of the OTIPM. As with the motor and process skills, I have modified the social interaction skills so that they can be used during informal, nonstandardized performance analyses. When they are scored according to the standardized criteria published in the AMPS (Fisher, 2006c), the School AMPS (Fisher et al., 2007), and the ESI (Fisher & Griswold, 2009) manuals, they become standardized performance analyses.

6.1 A Rationale for Documenting the Quality of Occupational Performance

Occupational therapists are accustomed to identifying a client's baseline level of ADL task performance based on the degree of independence with which the client performed the task. We are comfortable, therefore, using formal and informal rating scales that describe a client's level of independence in terms of the amount of physical assistance or verbal cues the client needs to perform various ADL tasks. However, many occupational therapists have expressed frustration with such scales because ***occupational therapy intervention is often directed toward improving the quality of a client's daily life task performance, and not solely toward increasing the client's level of independence***. That is, occupational therapists also consider the degree of physical effort, efficiency, and safety. When occupational therapists evaluate task performances that involve social interaction, they also consider the degree of observed social appropriateness. Finally, it is critical that we consider, where appropriate, the client's self-reported degree of satisfaction with relevant occupational performances.

It is critical, therefore, that we not restrict our descriptions of a client's daily life task performance to his or her overall level of independence; many of our clients achieve improved competence in performing daily life tasks which are not detected and/or documented when independence is the only criterion against which we evaluate their performance. Often, our clients demonstrate significantly less physical effort, become significantly more efficient, or become significantly safer, even when their level of need for assistance remains essentially unchanged. Others may not show improvements in quality of performance, but come to be more satisfied with what they are able to do.

I propose, therefore, that occupational therapists use six qualitative continua to document a client's daily life task performance. The six continua reflect the client's degree of (a) ***physical effort*** exerted during daily life task performance (i.e., the magnitude of observed physical difficulty or fatigue); (b) ***efficiency*** with which he or she carries out daily life tasks (i.e., the extent of observed disorganization or undesirable use of time, space, or objects); (c) ***safety*** when performing daily life tasks (i.e., the observed risk for personal injury or environmental damage); (d) ***independence*** when performing ADL tasks (i.e., the need for physical or verbal assistance; (e) ***social appropriateness*** during occupational performances that involve social interaction with others (i.e., observable social disruption, discomfort, immaturity, or awkwardness demonstrated or caused); and (f) ***satisfaction*** (i.e., verbalized satisfaction with daily life task performances).[32]

Before I present the six continua (see Section 6.5), I want to address the concerns that some therapists have expressed related to the qualitative nature of documenting a client's performance based on rating scales such as I present below. There are two important points I want to make:

---

[32] The occupational therapist may wish to add to this suggested list. For example, occupational therapists working with clients who experience pain or fatigue may choose to adapt the satisfaction scale to reflect degree of verbalized pain or fatigue.

1. ***There is a general misconception that ratings scales which describe a client's daily life task performance in terms of level of independence are objective.*** Whether level of independence (or need for assistance) is described by type of assistance (standby, verbal, physical), level of assistance (minimal, moderate, maximum), or amount of assistance (10% of the time, 25% of the time, 50% of the time), all of these scales are based on the ***subjective judgment*** of the person who makes the rating. While one can argue that we can observe and document that a person received standby assistance 10% of the time, we have to ask "Who was judging that the client needed assistance?" Another therapist may feel that the client did not need the assistance provided. Yet another therapist may have felt that the client needed minimal physical assistance and would have been more comfortable if the client had been given assistance 25% of the time.

   In actual practice, ***any rating scale that relies on professional judgment of a client's ADL performance is subjective.*** While the use of scales that reflect a client's level of independence is common and widely accepted as "objective," it is likely that ***we have confused (a) our familiarity with rating the client's level of independence, and (b) the common usage of these subjective scales with the idea that they are objective.***

2. ***While occupational therapists and other professionals sometimes express concerns about the subjective nature of an occupational therapist's professional (expert) judgment regarding a client's daily life task performance, the use of expert judgment is common.*** More important, there is evidence the ***interrater reliability of expert judgment is high*** (Shay et al., 1991; Weiler, Chiriboga, & Black, 1994; Whelihan, Lesher, Kleban, & Granick, 1984).

I feel, therefore, that it is imperative that occupational therapists (a) recognize the ***qualitative nature of all judgments***, (b) recognize that our judgments are ***no less valid or reliable*** than those made by other professionals or that are captured in ADL scales of independence, and (c) advocate for our need to more ***clearly document the quality of our clients' daily task performances using measureable, observable baselines, goals, and outcomes.*** In the following sections, I present taxonomies of motor, process, and social interaction skills (with their related ICF Activities and Participation codes (WHO, 2001) that have been shown to be helpful in evaluating and documenting the quality of the client's occupational performances.

6.2 Motor Skills

Observed actions that represent the quality of occupational performance as a person interacts with and moves task objects, and moves oneself around the task environment.

*Maria observed motor skills during a naturalistic and relevant daily life task performance when she saw Lars **reaching** for, grasping (**gripping**), and **lifting** a glass from the counter. She also observed motor skills when she observed him **manipulating** the knife as he repositioned it in his hand and altered his grasp before he started to spread butter on a slice of bread. Finally, she observed motor skills when she saw him **moving** the knife across the bread, and pressing downward (**calibrating**) with so much force that the bread tore.*

6.2.1 Body Position

STABILIZES — maintains an upright sitting or standing position while moving through the task environment or interacting with task objects such that there is no evidence of ***momentary*** propping or loss of balance that affects task performance (**d4153**, **d4154**).

Examples of ineffective skill include observations that the person (a) momentary stumbles while walking or interacting with task objects; (b) momentarily props on external supports when interacting with task objects, or (c) uses assistive devices (e.g., cane, rollator) while walking during task performance.

ALIGNS — sustains an upright sitting or standing position, as required during the task performance, such that there is no evidence of ***persistent*** propping, leaning, or loss of balance that affects the ongoing task performance (**d4153**, **d4154**).

Examples of ineffective skill include observations that the person persistently leans to the side, persistently props, or stands with a persistently stooped posture when interacting with task objects.

POSITIONS — positions body, arms, or wheelchair in relation to task objects (i.e., not too close or too far away) and as required for promoting the use of efficient arm movements during task performance (No parallel ICF code).

Examples of ineffective skill include observations that the person (a) uses awkward body or arm positions when picking up task objects ("elbow up"), or (b) positions the body or wheelchair too far from the counter so that it interferes with reaching for or placing tools or materials.

6.2.2 Obtaining and Holding Objects

REACHES — extends the arm, and when appropriate, bends the trunk, to effectively grasp or place task objects that are out of reach; includes skillfully using a reacher to obtain task objects (**d4452**).

Examples of ineffective skill include observations that the person demonstrates increased effort when reaching for or placing task objects.

BENDS — actively flexes, rotates, or twists the trunk in a manner and direction appropriate to the task, as when bending to pick up a task object from the floor or to sit down in a chair or on a bed (**d4105, d4104**).

Examples of ineffective skill include observations that the person has (a) increased effort or stiffness when bending to reach task objects, or (b) increased effort or stiffness when bending to sit down.

GRIPS — pinches or grasps task objects such that the task object does not slip (e.g., from the person's fingers or hand, from between the teeth) (**d4400, d4401**).

Examples of ineffective skill include observations that the person has a "grip slip" on a task object held in the person's hand or between two body parts (e.g., knees).

MANIPULATES — uses dexterous grasp and release patterns, isolated finger movements, and coordinated in-hand manipulation patterns when interacting with small task objects (e.g., difficulty manipulating buttons when buttoning, difficulty using isolated finger movements to open and close scissors when cutting) (**d4402**).

Examples of ineffective skill include observations that the person has decreased dexterity or fumbles during manipulation of task objects (e.g., knife, pencil).

COORDINATES — uses two or more body parts together to stabilize and manipulate task objects during bilateral motor tasks, such as when holding paper in one hand when cutting with scissors held in the other hand, or holding a jar between the knees when removing the lid (no parallel ICF code; do ***not*** confuse with Person factors and body functions code **b7602**).

Examples of ineffective skill include observations that the person (a) has a "grip slip" or fumbles task objects when using two hands, or (b) has a "grip slip" of a task object stabilized under one hand (e.g., bread, paper) while interacting with the task object with another body part (e.g., spreading butter, cutting with scissors).

6.2.3 Moving Self and Objects

MOVES — pushes or pulls task objects along a supporting surface, pulls to open or pushes to close doors and drawers, or pushes on wheels to propel a wheelchair (**d4450**, **d4451**).

Examples of ineffective skill include observations that the person (a) becomes unstable and/or needs to prop on external objects when opening doors or drawers, (b) demonstrates increased effort when pushing or pulling task objects (e.g., sliding a book across a desk, pulling a sleeve up the arm), or (c) demonstrates increased effort when propelling the wheelchair.

LIFTS — raises or lifts task objects; includes lifting an object from one place to another, but without ambulating or moving from one place to another (**d4300**).

Examples of ineffective skill include observations that the person (a) uses two hands to lift small or lightweight task objects, (b) uses increased effort when lifting task objects, or (c) slides task objects that typically are lifted.

WALKS — ambulates on level surfaces and changes direction while walking without shuffling the feet, lurching, instability, propping, or using assistive devices (e.g., cane, walker, wheelchair) during the task performance (**d450**, especially **d4500**).

Examples of ineffective skill include observations that the person (a) walks with some unsteadiness and/or holds on to the counter or furniture to maintain stability while walking; (b) uses a wheelchair throughout task performance, or (c) uses assistive devices (e.g., cane, rollator) while walking during task performance.

TRANSPORTS — carries task objects from one place to another while walking, moving in a wheelchair, or using a walker (**d4301**, **d4302**, **d4303**, **d4304**).

Examples of ineffective skill include observations that the person (a) is unstable when transporting objects, (b) slides or lifts objects that typically are transported, or (c) has difficulty transporting objects in the wheelchair.

CALIBRATES — regulates or grades the force, speed, and extent of movements when interacting with task objects (e.g., not too much nor too little — not crushing task objects, not banging a task object when placing it on a table, pushing a door with enough force that it closes) (no parallel ICF code; do ***not*** confuse with Person factors and body functions codes **b760** or **b765**).

Examples of ineffective skill include observations that the person (a) exerts too much pressure such that a task object is crushed, (b) exerts too little force such that a door does not close, (c) bangs objects when placing them on the counter, or (d) reaches too far or too fast such that a task object is knocked over or onto the floor.

FLOWS — uses smooth and fluid arm and wrist movements when interacting with task objects (no parallel ICF code; do ***not*** confuse with Person factors and body functions codes **b7650** or **b7651**).

Examples of ineffective skill include observations that the person demonstrates jerky or stiff arm or wrist movements when interacting with task objects.

6.2.4 Sustaining Performance

ENDURES — persists and completes the task without ***obvious*** evidence of physical fatigue, pausing to rest, or stopping to "catch ones breath" (no parallel ICF code; do not confuse with Person factors and body functions code **b445** as the focus of Endures is not on underlying respiratory or cardiovascular capacity).

Examples of ineffective skill include observations that the person (a) pauses to rest because of physical fatigue, (b) has shortness of breath during task performance, or (c) demonstrates labored breathing during task performance.

PACES — maintains a consistent and effective rate or tempo of performance throughout the performance of actions and steps of the entire task (**d2100, d2101, d2200, d2201, d2302**).

Examples of ineffective skill include observations that the person (a) proceeds too quickly, (b) proceeds too slowly, or (c) demonstrates an uneven pace.

(*Note*. Paces is both a motor skill and a process skill, but we score it only once, based on the person's overall rate or tempo of performance.)

6.3 Process Skills

Observed actions that represent the quality of occupational performance as a person (a) selects, interacts with, and uses task tools and materials; (b) carries out individual actions and steps; and (c) modifies performance when problems are encountered.

> *Maria observed process skills during a naturalistic and relevant daily life task performance when she saw Lars* ***choose*** *the butter and whole grain bread, and when he paused before he* ***initiated*** *buttering the bread. She also observed a process skill as he watched Lars* ***continue*** *spreading, without taking any pauses.*

6.3.1 Sustaining Performance

PACES — maintains a consistent and effective rate or tempo of performance throughout the performance of actions and steps of the entire task (**d2100, d2101, d2200, d2201, d2302**).

Examples of ineffective skill include observations that the person (a) proceeds too quickly, (b) proceeds too slowly, or (c) demonstrates an uneven pace.

(*Note*. Paces is both a motor skill and a process skill, but we score it only once, based on the person's overall rate or tempo of performance.)

ATTENDS — maintains focus on the task performance such that the person does not look away from what he or she is doing (e.g., toward extraneous auditory or visual stimuli), thus interrupting the ongoing task progression (**d160**).

Examples of ineffective skill include observations that the person looks away from what he or she is doing and this interrupts with the task progression.

HEEDS — uses goal-directed task actions that are focused toward carrying out and completing a specified task (i.e., the outcome originally agreed on or specified by another), and using task materials that were specified (e.g., making brewed coffee, not instant coffee, if the client specified that he or she would make brewed coffee; writing sentences with a pencil, not a marker, if the students' teacher specified that they were to write with pencils); does ***not*** include restoration of task objects (possibly **d210**, but **d210** is more vague in that it only includes carrying out and completing a task).

Examples of ineffective skill include observations that the person (a) performs a task different from what was specified (e.g., makes a salad, but omits a specified ingredient; does not color all the shapes on the specified workbook page), or (b) completes the task using materials different from those specified (e.g., makes instant coffee instead of the specified brewed coffee, colors with markers when crayons were specified).

6.3.2 Applying Knowledge

CHOOSES — selects necessary and appropriate type and number of tools and materials for the task; includes choosing the tools and materials that the person specified he or she would use prior to the initiation of the task (no parallel ICF code, but choosing needed task objects can be viewed as an undefined element of **d210**).

Examples of ineffective skill include observations that the person (a) chooses incorrect items, (b) chooses too many items, or (c) does not choose needed items.

USES — employs tools and materials (a) as they are intended (e.g., using a knife to cut or spread, but not to stir foods; using a pencil sharpener to sharpen a pencil, but not to sharpen a crayon), and (b) in a reasonable (including hygienic) fashion, given their intrinsic properties and the availability (or lack of availability) of other objects (no parallel ICF code, but using needed task objects appropriately can be viewed as an undefined element of **d210**).

Examples of ineffective skill include observations that the person (a) uses a task object for an inappropriate purpose (e.g., uses shaving cream to brush the teeth), or (b) uses an object in an unsanitary manner (e.g., completely licks the knife clean and then puts it back into the jelly jar).

HANDLES — supports, stabilizes, and holds tools and materials in an appropriate manner, protecting them from damage, slipping, moving, or falling (no parallel ICF code, but handling task objects appropriately can be viewed as an undefined element of **d210**).

Examples of ineffective skill include observations that the person (a) delays stabilizing a task object, (b) holds task objects in a manner that is awkward, or (c) allows an object to tilt or fall because it was not adequately supported.

INQUIRES — (a) seeks needed verbal or written information by asking questions or reading directions or labels, and (b) does not ask for information in situations where the person has been fully oriented to the task and environment and had immediate prior awareness of the answer (e.g., asking where task tools or materials are located after having just placed them where he or she wanted them); does ***not*** pertain to asking for help (**d166** [reading directions or labels]; asking questions has no parallel ICF code, but can be viewed as an undefined element of **d350**).

Examples of ineffective skill include observations that the person (a) asks questions related to information that was discussed and clarified before beginning the task performance, or (b) demonstrates delays reading needed written information.

6.3.3 Temporal Organization

INITIATES — starts or begins ***the next*** action or step without hesitation; does ***not*** include having to complete the action or step (**d210**, but **d210** places the emphasis on initiating the overall task, not the individual actions or steps that comprise the task).

Examples of ineffective skill include observations that the person pauses before beginning the next action or step of the task performance.

CONTINUES — performs single sustained actions or a series of step actions (e.g., cutting actions when slicing a carrot, erasing actions when erasing a mistake, letter writing actions when writing a word) without interruptions or pauses such that once an action or task step is initiated, the individual continues on until the action or step is completed (no parallel ICF code, but continuing action without interruption can be viewed as a component of sustaining a task, **d210**, or as part of carrying out simple or complex and coordinated actions of integrated or complex tasks, **d220**).

Examples of ineffective skill include observations that the person (a) begins an action sequence or step and then pauses before going on to complete the action or step; or (b) starts an action sequence or step, stops and does something else, and then goes back to performing the original action sequence or step.

SEQUENCES — performs steps in an effective or logical order for efficient use of time and energy; and with an absence of (a) randomness or lack of logic in the ordering, and/or (b) inappropriate repetition of steps (no parallel ICF code, but sequencing task steps appropriately can be viewed as a component of sustaining a task, **d210**, or as part of carrying out simple or complex and coordinated actions of integrated or complex tasks, **d220**).

Examples of ineffective skill include observations that the person performs steps in an order that is clearly "strange" or illogical (e.g., cuts out an intricate figure and then colors it, causing the figure to wrinkle; puts on a blouse and then puts on underwear).

TERMINATES — brings to completion single actions or single steps without inappropriate persistence (i.e., continues to perform the action or step beyond what is needed or required), or premature cessation (i.e., stops performing the action or step before it is completed); does ***not*** pertain to restoration (no parallel ICF code, but terminating single actions and single steps can be viewed as a component of sustaining a task, **d210**, or as part of carrying out simple or complex and coordinated actions of integrated or complex tasks, **d220**).

Examples of ineffective skill include observations that the person (a) performs an action too long (e.g., spreads and spreads the glue on the paper), or (b) stops an action too soon (e.g., does not mix the mayonnaise thoroughly into the tuna).

6.3.4 Organizing Space and Objects

SEARCHES/LOCATES — looks for and locates tools and materials in a logical manner, both within and beyond the immediate environment; includes not asking where task objects are located before looking for them, provided the person was aware prior to beginning the task where tools and materials are located (no parallel ICF code, but searching for and finding task objects can be viewed as a component of preparing and organizing materials, **d210**).

Examples of ineffective skill include observations that the person (a) looks in more than one place before finding a task object, or (b) asks where task objects are located before looking for them even though the person was aware prior to beginning the task where tools and materials are located.

GATHERS — collects together needed or misplaced tools and materials, including (a) collecting related tools and materials into the same workspace; and (b) collecting and replacing materials that have spilled, fallen, or been misplaced (no parallel ICF code, but gathering task objects can be viewed as a component of preparing and organizing materials, **d210**).

Examples of ineffective skill include observations that the person (a) does not gather related task objects into the same workspace, or (b) delays wiping up or regathering objects that spill or fall on the floor.

ORGANIZES — logically positions or spatially arranges tools and materials in an orderly fashion (a) within a single workspace, and (b) between multiple appropriate workspaces, in order to facilitate ease of task performance (e.g., the workspace is not too spread out or too crowded); includes spatially arranging clothing such as when getting dressed or ironing (no parallel ICF code, but organizing task objects within and between workspaces can be viewed as a component of organizing space and materials, **d210**).

Examples of ineffective skill include observations that the person (a) has a workspace that is too crowded, (b) has related task objects spread out into two or more workspaces, or (c) has difficulty spatially arranging clothing in order to put it on.

RESTORES — (a) puts away tools and materials in appropriate places, (b) restores immediate workspace(s) to original condition (e.g., wiping work surface clean, putting tools and materials away in cupboards or drawers), (c) closes and seals containers and coverings when indicated, and (d) saves work on a computer before exiting the program (no parallel ICF code, but restoring task objects appropriately can be viewed as an undefined element of **d210**).

Examples of ineffective skill include observations that the person (a) does not put away tools and materials when done, (b) does not wipe or pick up objects that have spilled or fallen on the floor, or (c) does not close open containers (e.g., glue bottle, bread bag).

NAVIGATES — modifies the movement pattern of the arm, body, or wheelchair to maneuver around obstacles that are encountered in the course of moving through space, such that undesirable contact with obstacles (e.g., knocking over, bumping into) is avoided; includes holding and maneuvering objects around obstacles (no parallel ICF code, but navigating the body or body parts around obstacles can be viewed as an undefined element of **d210**). (*Note.* Navigates should be viewed as a skill related to organizing oneself in space, not a skill related to mobility.)

Examples of ineffective skill include observations that the person (a) bumps his or her body or hand into task objects, or (b) bumps the wheelchair into furniture or walls.

6.3.5 Adapting Performance

NOTICES/RESPONDS — responds appropriately to (a) nonverbal task-related cues (e.g., task object rolling, appliance heating, liquid dripping) that provide feedback regarding task progression, (b) the spatial arrangement of objects to one another (e.g., alignment of objects during stacking, alignment of numbers on a page), and (c) cupboard doors or drawers that have been left open during the task performance. Notices and, when indicated, makes an effective and efficient response (no parallel ICF code; noticing and responding to task-related cues is related to modification of one's task performance to prevent or correct errors, possibly an undefined adaptation element in **d2**).

Examples of ineffective skill include observations that the person (a) does not notice/respond to an appliance that is not working (e.g., iron not heating, vacuum not "sucking"), (b) does not notice/respond to liquid that is dripping or spilling, or (c) does not notice/respond when number columns are not aligned on the page.

ADJUSTS — changes working environments in anticipation of, or in response to, problems that arise; anticipates or responds to problems effectively by making some change (a) between workspaces by moving to a new workspace or bringing in or removing tools and materials from the present workspace, or (b) in an environmental condition (e.g., turning on or off the tap, turning up or down the temperature) (no parallel ICF code; adjusting by changing the working environment is related to modification of one's task performance to prevent or correct errors, possibly an undefined adaptation element in **d2**).

Examples of ineffective skill include observations that the person (a) delays moving task objects to a new workplace in order to overcome a problem; (b) repeatedly and unnecessarily turns switches on or off, adjusts the volume on a radio, or turns a dial on a stove; or (c) delays turning electrical appliances on or off.

ACCOMMODATES — modifies actions or the location of objects within the workspace, in anticipation of, or in response to, problems that might arise; anticipates or responds to problems effectively by (a) changing the method with which one is performing an action sequence, (b) changing the manner in which one interacts with or handles tools and materials already in the workspace, and (c) asking for assistance when appropriate or needed (no parallel ICF code; accommodating by changing how one interacts with task objects is related to modification of one's task performance to prevent or correct errors, possibly an undefined adaptation element in **d2**).

Examples of ineffective skill include observations that the person (a) delays changing the way he or she interacts with task objects in order to correct a problem, or (b) does not change his or her actions to prevent problems with any of the other performance skills.

BENEFITS — anticipates and prevents undesirable circumstances or problems from recurring or persisting; includes responding appropriately to verbal cues intended to lead to correction of errors (no parallel ICF code; benefiting such that problems in performance do not recur or persist is related to modification of one's task performance to prevent or correct errors, possibly an undefined adaptation element in **d2**).

Examples of ineffective skill include observations that the person (a) demonstrates performance skill problems that recur or persist, (b) repeats an action or step for no apparent reason (e.g., to correct a problem) and that delays the task progression, or (c) delays responding appropriately to verbal cues.

6.4 Social Interaction Skills

Observed actions that represent the quality of occupational performance as a person communicates and interacts with others during task performances that involve social interaction.

> *James observed social interaction skills when he observed Jennifer* ***look*** at and ***turn toward*** *her social partner. He also observed social interaction skills as Jennifer* ***gestured*** *and* ***produced speech****. Finally, James observed a social interaction skill when he saw Jennifer interrupt her social partner* ***(timing response)****.*

6.4.1 Initiating and Terminating Social Interaction

APPROACHES/STARTS — uses strategies appropriate to the social context to approach and initiate interaction with the social partner; includes catching the attention of the social partner through (a) asking a question or (b) sending a greeting or introductory phrase to initiate a social interaction (e.g., "Hello," "Excuse me," "Can I interrupt you?"); also includes responding to the arrival or greeting from the social partner (**d3500**).

Examples of ineffective skill include observations that the person (a) uses socially inappropriate methods of catching the attention of the social partner; (b) initiates a social interaction without a preliminary greeting, when a greeting would have been appropriate, or (c) responds to a social partner's initiation of the social interaction with an inappropriate response.

CONCLUDES/DISENGAGES — terminates the conversation or social interaction using customary termination statements, brings to closure the topic under discussion, and disengages or says goodbye using appropriate phrases and ceremonies, as appropriate to the context and degree of familiarity with the social partner; includes the ability to send verbal and nonverbal messages that termination is desired, and then using appropriate strategies to carry the termination of the conversation or social interaction through to an appropriate end (**d3502**).

Examples of ineffective skill include observations that the person (a) delays ending the social interaction by unnecessarily extending the conversation, (b) ends the social interaction in a manner that is somewhat abrupt, or (c) ends the social interaction in a manner such that the social partner is unclear that the interaction has ended.

6.4.2 Producing Social Interaction

PRODUCES SPEECH — produces spoken, signed, or augmentative (i.e., computer-generated) messages with literal meaning; includes producing clearly articulated speech that is audible and expresses meaning, given the social context (**d330**, **d340**, **d3601**, **d3350**).

Examples of ineffective skill include observations that the person (a) produces speech that is barely audible or not clearly articulated (e.g., mumbling), or (b) produces poorly articulated signs.

GESTICULATES — uses socially appropriate gestures to communicate or support a message (e.g., shaking one's head, frowning, smiling, waving one's hand) to send signals to the social partner (**d3350**).

Examples of ineffective skill include observations that the person (a) uses gestures that are not relevant to the social context; (b) uses gestures whose meaning, given the social context, remains unclear; (c) sends gestures that are exaggerated or delayed; or (d) uses socially inappropriate methods to gesture to a social partner.

SPEAKS FLUENTLY — speaks in a fluent and continuous manner with an even flow (not too fast, not too slow); includes speaking without pauses or delays ***during*** spoken, signed, or augmentative (i.e., computer-generated) message (no parallel ICF code; do not confuse with Person factors and body functions codes **b3300** or **b3301**).

Examples of ineffective skill include observations that the person (a) speaks in a hesitant manner (e.g., with short pauses, stuttering), (b) speaks in a manner that is monotonous, or (c) speaks too fast or too slow, or with an uneven tempo (sometimes fast, sometimes slow).

6.4.3 Physically Supporting Social Interaction

TURNS TOWARD — actively positions or turns the body and the face toward the social partner or the person who is speaking (no parallel ICF code).

Examples of ineffective skill include observations that the person (a) does not turn the body and/or face toward the social partner, (b) delays turning to face the social partner, or (c) turns body away from social partner.

LOOKS — makes eye contact with the social partner in a manner that is relaxed; includes adjusting the frequency and duration of eye contact to match that of the social partner (no parallel ICF code).

Examples of ineffective skill include observations that the person (a) looks down or away from social partner when interacting, (b) delays looking at the social partner, or (c) maintains eye contact for a period of time that is too short or too long.

PLACES SELF — places oneself at an appropriate distance from the social partner during the social interaction and as appropriate, given the social context and the degree of familiarity with the social partner; implies acting according to the social partner's cues about personal space, and adjusting one's distance to the type of social interaction and degree of familiarity with the social partner (**d7204**).

Examples of ineffective skill include observations that the person (a) places him- or herself (including hands or feet) too close to the social partner, or (b) places him- or herself at a distance that is too far from the social partner.

TOUCHES — responds to and uses touch or bodily contact with the social partner in a manner that is socially appropriate (**d7105**).

Examples of ineffective skill include observations that the person (a) repeatedly bumps, touches, or kicks the social partner; (b) avoids touching or being touched when it is appropriate, socially and culturally relevant, and "natural" (e.g., pulling away from the touch); or (c) touches the social partner to an extent or in a manner that is inappropriate for the context or relationship of people (e.g., hugging an unfamiliar social partner).

REGULATES — controls impulses and behaviors that are not part of communication and not appropriate to the social situation; includes assuming body positions that are appropriate to the type of social interaction and degree of familiarity with the social partner (**d7202**).

Examples of ineffective skill include observations that the person (a) demonstrates repetitive hand or body movements (e.g., twisting hands, drumming fingers, clicking pens, chewing gum); (b) assumes a position that is sexually provocative; (c) positions him- or herself slumped down in the chair or half lying on the table; (d) uses repetitive nonsense verbalization (e.g., noises such as "ta, ta, ta, ta" or phrases such as "don't know, don't know, don't know"); or (e) uses swear words or speaks with a loud voice.

6.4.4 Shaping Content of Social Interaction

QUESTIONS — requests relevant facts and information, or ask questions that support the intended purpose of the social interaction (e.g., asking questions in order to seek socially-relevant information about the social partner's opinions, interests, or needs; asking questions needed to manage a task) (no parallel ICF code).

Examples of ineffective skill include observations that the person (a) asks for inappropriate personal information; (b) asks questions, when information is known or has just been clearly stated; (c) asks an irrelevant question; or (d) delays to ask a question.

REPLIES — keeps conversation going by replying to questions and comments that are appropriate to the social context; includes providing information and/or opinions when asked for them; also includes giving a relevant reply to an apology or feedback expressed by the social partner or elaborating on the ideas being discussed (**d3501**).

Examples of ineffective skill include observations that the person (a) replies with a response that has too little or too much detail; (b) replies with a response that is irrelevant; (c) sends a message that is indirect or circuitous; or (d) does not reply to a question, a comment, an apology, or feedback received from the social partner.

DISCLOSES — shares information, opinions, and feelings about oneself or others in an appropriate manner, given the social context and degree of familiarity with the social partner; implies sharing at a level that corresponds to the social partner's degree of openness, provided that level is also appropriate; includes, when socially appropriate, revealing personal information in a gradual, step by step manner that matches the social partner's level of disclosure (**d710**).

Examples of ineffective skill include observations that the person (a) discloses personal information or opinions that are inappropriate, given the situation and level of familiarity with the social partner; (b) discloses somewhat inappropriate personal information about others; (c) reveals too much personal information, too soon (d) expresses negative and/or belittling feelings about oneself or others; or (e) expresses elevated opinion of oneself (e.g., bragging).

EXPRESSES EMOTIONS — displays affect and emotions in a way that is socially acceptable, and appropriate to the context and the level of familiarity with the social partner; includes expressing emotion through one's facial expression or tone of voice in a manner that matches the message sent; also includes expressing emotion both as a listener and as a speaker (**d7202**).

Examples of ineffective skill include observations that the person (a) smiles or giggles when nervous or uncertain, or without visible cause; (b) expresses emotion that does not match spoken message (e.g., smiling when talking about someone's grief); (c) uses sarcasm or a tone of voice that does not match the message being sent; or (d) demonstrates minimal emotion (e.g., flat affect).

DISAGREES — expresses differences of opinion in a socially appropriate manner and as appropriate to the social context and degree of familiarity with the social partner (**d7103**).

Examples of ineffective skill include observations that the person (a) comments on the social partner's stated opinions in a manner that is defensive or argumentative, (b) does not respond to the social partner's suggestion (e.g., "Shall we try this approach?")

or opinion (e.g., "I think that we should give him another chance."), or (c) expresses a difference in opinion by whining.

THANKS — uses appropriate words, phrases, gestures, and ceremonies to confirm receipt of services, offers, gifts, and/or compliments; includes expressing gratitude for the generosity or kindness shown by the social partner or showing conventional courtesy in the context of economical transactions involving goods and services (no parallel ICF code).

Examples of ineffective skill include observations that the person (a) uses socially undesirable methods to express gratitude or thanks, (b) says, "Thank you" sarcastically, or (c) does not say, "Thank you" when socially indicated.

6.4.5 Maintaining Flow of Social Interaction

TRANSITIONS — smoothly transitions the conversation to a closely related topic, and/or changes the topic without disrupting the conversation (**d3501**).

Examples of ineffective skill include observations that the person (a) abruptly transitions to a new topic that is irrelevant to the ongoing conversation and intended purpose of the social interaction; (b) persists in discussing the same or an earlier topic after the conversation has transitioned on to a new one; or (c) repeatedly asks the same question, interfering with transition to a new topic.

TIMES RESPONSE — replies to social messages without delay or hesitation, or without interrupting the social partner (no parallel ICF code).

Examples of ineffective skill include observations that the person (a) interrupts the social partner before he or she has completed his or her message, (b) answers the social partner's question before the social partner has finished asking it, (c) delays responding to the social partner's message and/or to take one's own turn, or (d) does not reply to a question or comment received from the social partner.

TIMES DURATION — speaks for reasonable time periods that are appropriate, given the social partner and the context; includes adjusting the length of one's turn, depending on the situation and the complexity of the message (no parallel ICF code).

Examples of ineffective skill include observations that the person (a) prolongs message beyond that needed to communicate the desired information; (b) sends short, one to two word messages, when social context would expect longer messages; or (c) does not complete a message, resulting in message "hanging in the air" and disruption of the quality of social interaction.

TAKES TURNS — takes one's turn and gives the social partner the freedom to take his or her turn; includes sending cues or messages that signal whose turn it is to send a message; also includes not allowing oneself to be dominated by others (**d3501**).

Examples of ineffective skill include observations that the person (a) dominates the social interaction; (b) lets him- or herself be dominated by the social partner; (c) asks several questions in rapid succession, without waiting for replies; or (d) makes a suggestion and then continues the conversation without waiting for a reply.

6.4.6 Verbally Supporting Social Interaction

MATCHES LANGUAGE — uses a tone of voice, dialect, and level of language that is appropriate to the situation and the social partner's abilities and level of understanding; implies varying one's level of language according to (a) the type of social interaction (e.g., formal speech vs. casual conversation), (b) the level of language used by the social partner (e.g., that of a child vs. that of an adult; use of dialect or jargon), and (c) the intended purpose of the social interaction and degree of familiarity with the social partner (no parallel ICF code).

Examples of ineffective skill include observations that the person (a) uses childlike language, or phrases that are typical of a teenager, with an adult social partner; (b) uses words that are too simple or too sophisticated, given the social partner's age or status; (c) uses slang or jargon; (d) uses a highly pitched, childlike voice with an adult social partner; or (e) whines when responding to the social partner.

CLARIFIES — ensures, in a manner appropriate to the social context and the degree of familiarity with the social partner, that the social partner is "following" the conversation or social interaction; includes recognizing when the social partner does not comprehend or understand a message and then responding appropriately by clarifying or giving an explanation (no parallel ICF code).

Examples of ineffective skill include observations that the person (a) clarifies unnecessarily (e.g., clarifies some messages that were clear and that the social partner acknowledged receiving), (b) does not respond by clarifying when the social partner sends a message that he or she needs clarification (e.g., asks the social partner to clarify, displays facial expression of confusion), or (c) verifies unnecessarily that the social partner has understood (e.g., repeatedly asking, “Do you understand?”, “Do you understand?”).

ACKNOWLEDGES/ENCOURAGES — acknowledges receipt of messages and/or encourages the social partner to continue interaction by nodding, using facial expressions (e.g., smiling), gesturing, or verbalizing encouraging statements (e.g., “Um-huh,” “Good point”) (no parallel ICF code).

Examples of ineffective skill include observations that the person (a) nods or smiles, even when messages are not being sent; or (b) does not send messages to encourage the social partner to continue social interaction, when dong so is socially indicated.

EMPATHIZES — expresses a supportive attitude towards the social partner by agreeing with, empathizing with, or expressing understanding of the social partner’s feelings and experiences; includes using gestures of concern (e.g., hugging, patting the social partner on the back) as appropriate, given the social context and degree of familiarity with the social partner (no parallel ICF code).

Examples of ineffective skill include observations that the person (a) does not send messages of support for the social partner’s experience or feelings (including implicit messages requesting emotional support), when the need to send a message was clearly indicated; or (b) delays sending messages of support for the social partner’s experience or feelings.

6.4.7 Adapting Social Interaction

(*Note*. The following skills are based on the process skills presented above, but have been modified for use in the evaluation of task performances involving social interaction.)

HEEDS — uses goal-directed social interactions that are focused toward carrying out and completing the intended purpose of the social interaction (no parallel ICF code).

Examples of ineffective skill include observations that the person (a) engages in a social interaction that has a different intended purpose than originally specified (e.g., engaging in some “small talk” during a problem-solving task; sometimes playing rather than collaboratively working on a project), (b) engages in a social interaction with another person who is not part of the intended social interaction (e.g., talking on a telephone), (c) asks questions or makes comments that are irrelevant to the intended social interaction, or (d) transitions to a new topic that is somewhat irrelevant to the ongoing conversation and intended purpose of the social interaction, disrupting the intended purpose of the social interaction.

ACCOMMODATES — modifies his or her social interaction in anticipation of, or in response to, problems that might arise; includes apologizing or excusing oneself, when socially indicated. The person anticipates or responds to problems effectively by (a) changing the method with which he or she is interacting, or (b) asking for assistance when appropriate or needed (no parallel ICF code).

Examples of ineffective skill include observations that the person (a) asks for help that is inappropriate or not needed, (b) delays to ask for help, (c) delays sending a message of apology after unexpectedly burping, or (d) demonstrates any other social interaction skill deficit.

BENEFITS — anticipates and prevents undesirable circumstances or problems in the social interaction from recurring or persisting; includes responding appropriately to verbal cues intended to lead to correction of inappropriate social interaction (no parallel ICF code).

Examples of ineffective skill include observations that the person (a) repeats words or sentences unnecessarily; (b) delays before responding appropriately to a verbal cue, interrupting the progression of the social interaction; or (c) demonstrates persistence or recurrence of a social skill deficit.

6.5 Nonstandardized Scoring Criteria

6.5.1 Occupational Performance — Effort

Our judgment of a person's level of effort is based on the degree of ***observed physical effort***, ***clumsiness***, or ***fatigue*** the person demonstrates during the performance of a daily life task. The judgment is primarily based on the person's performance on the ***motor skills*** as they were manifested during the occupational performance.

Increase in Effort — ***Physical Effort, Clumsiness, or Fatigue***

No increase: Person demonstrated ***no*** physical effort, clumsiness, or fatigue

Minimal: Person demonstrated a ***mild*** degree of physical effort, clumsiness, or fatigue

Moderate: Person demonstrated a ***modest*** degree of physical effort, clumsiness, or fatigue

Marked: Person demonstrated a ***substantial*** degree of physical effort, clumsiness, or fatigue; ***or*** entered into, but was ***unable to complete the task***

6.5.2 Occupational Performance — Efficiency

Our judgment of a person's overall efficiency is based on the ***degree of observed disorganization***, or ***inappropriate use of time, space, or objects*** the person demonstrated during the occupational performance. The judgment is primarily based on the person's performance on the ***process skills*** as they were manifested during the task performance.

Decrease in Efficiency — *Disorganization or Undesirable Use of Time, Space, or Objects*

Efficient: Person demonstrated ***no*** disorganization or undesirable use of time, space, or objects

Minimal: Person demonstrated a ***mild*** degree of disorganization or undesirable use of time, space, or objects

Moderate: Person demonstrated a ***modest*** degree of disorganization or undesirable use of time, space, or objects

Marked: Person demonstrated a ***substantial*** degree of disorganization or undesirable use of time, space, or objects; ***or*** entered into, but was ***unable to complete the task***

6.5.3 Occupational Performance — Safety

Our judgment of a person's safety during occupational performance is based on the person's ***observed risk to injure him- or herself*** or ***cause damage to the environment*** as manifested during the person's task performance. All ***motor and process skills*** are considered in the formulation of this judgment. We only consider, however, what we observed as unsafe performance during the daily life task observed. We do not base our judgment on what we think ***might occur*** in the future. This does not mean that the occupational therapist cannot also use the following criteria to judge a person's ***overall level*** of safety.

Decrease in safety — ***Risk for Personal Injury or Environmental Damage***

Safe: Person demonstrated ***no*** risk for personal injury or environmental damage

Minimal: Person demonstrated a ***mild*** degree of risk for personal injury or environmental damage

Moderate: Person demonstrated a ***modest*** degree of risk for personal injury or environmental damage

Marked: Person demonstrated a ***substantial*** degree of risk for personal injury or environmental damage; an ***imminent risk*** for personal injury or environmental damage ***occurred during*** the task performance; ***or*** entered into, but was ***unable to safely complete the task***

6.5.4 Occupational Performance — Need for Assistance or Support Provided

Our judgment of the level of ***observed*** physical or verbal assistance a person receives during the performance of a task is based on the ***frequency of the assistance*** (e.g., how often the therapist provided assistance) rather than the intensity of the assistance (i.e., the degree of physical effort a therapist exerted when he or she provided assistance). All of the ***motor, process, and social interaction skills*** are considered in the formulation of this judgment.

Frequency of assistance provided — ***Physical or verbal assistance***

Independent: Person received ***no*** need physical or verbal assistance

Occasional: Person received ***occasional or intermittent*** verbal or physical assistance

Frequent: Person received ***frequent*** verbal or physical assistance

Constant: Person received ***constant*** verbal or physical assistance; ***or*** entered into, but was ***unable to complete the task without constant assistance***

6.5.5 Occupational performance — Social Appropriateness

Our judgment of a person's overall level of social appropriateness is based on the degree of ***observable social immaturity***, or ***disruption, discomfort, and/or awkwardness*** demonstrated or caused during occupational performances that involve social interaction with others. The judgment is primarily based on the person's performance on the ***social interaction skills*** as they were manifested during the performance of tasks involving social interaction with others. Such tasks can be related to ADL, work, or play and leisure, and they may or may not be primarily social in nature.

Lack of social appropriateness — *Disruption, disturbance, immaturity of social interaction*

Appropriate: Person demonstrated and/or caused ***no*** immaturity, or disruption or disturbance of the social interaction

Minimal*:** Person demonstrated some immaturity, or demonstrated and/or caused a ***mild degree of disruption or disturbance of the social interaction

Moderate*:** Person demonstrated moderate immaturity, or demonstrated and/or caused a ***modest degree of disruption or disturbance of the social interaction

Marked: Person demonstrated marked immaturity, or demonstrated and/or caused a ***substantial*** disruption or disturbance of the social interaction; ***or*** entered into, but was ***unable to complete the social interaction task***

6.5.6 Occupational performance — Satisfaction

Our judgment of a person's overall level of ***satisfaction with occupational performance*** is based on the person's verbalizations. The judgment is primarily based on the person's self-report, but self-reports of others in the person constellation may also be considered.

Limited satisfaction — *Verbalizations of dissatisfaction*

Satisfied: Person verbalized ***no*** dissatisfaction and/or verbalized satisfaction

Minimal*:** Person verbalized some or a ***mild degree of dissatisfaction

Moderate*:** Person verbalized moderate or a ***modest degree of dissatisfaction

Marked: Person verbalized marked or a ***substantial*** degree of dissatisfaction; ***or*** entered into, but ***did not complete the task because of extreme dissatisfaction***

7. REFERENCES

American Occupational Therapy Association (1993). Position paper: Purposeful activity. *American Journal of Occupational Therapy, 47,* 1081-1082.

American Occupational Therapy Association (2002). Occupational therapy practice framework: Domain and process. *American Journal of Occupational Therapy, 56*, 609-639.

American Occupational Therapy Association (2005). *Occupational therapy code of ethics (2005).* Retrieved September 3, 2007 from http//www.aota.org/Practioners/Ethics/Docs/Standards/38527.aspx.

American Occupational Therapy Association (2008). Occupational therapy practice framework: Domain and process (2nd ed.). *American Journal of Occupational Therapy, 62*, 625-683.

Benedict, R. H. B., Harris, A. E., Markow, T., McCormick, J. A., Nuechterlein, K. H., & Asarnow, R. F. (1994). Effects of attention training on information processing in schizophrenia. *Schizophrenia Bulletin, 20,* 537-546.

Bernspång, B., Asplund, K., Eriksson, S., & Fugl-Meyer, A. R. (1987). Motor and perceptual impairments in acute stroke patients: Effects on self-care ability. *Stroke, 18*, 1081-1086.

Bowen, R. E. (1996). The Issue Is — Should occupational therapy adopt a consumer-based model of service delivery? *American Journal of Occupational Therapy, 50,* 899-902.

Bracciano, A. G. (2008). In M. V. Radomski & C. A. Trombly Latham (Eds.), *Occupational therapy for physical dysfunction* (6th ed.) (pp. 542-571). Philadelphia: Lippincott Williams & Wilkins.

Bruce, M. A., & Borg, B. (2002). *Psychosocial occupational therapy: Core for occupation-based practice* (3nd ed.). Thorofare, NJ: Slack.

Canadian Association of Occupational Therapists. (1997). *Enabling occupation: An occupational therapy perspective.* Ottawa, ON: CAOT Publications ACE.

Canadian Association of Occupational Therapists. (2002). *Enabling occupation: An occupational therapy perspective* (revised ed.). Ottawa, ON: CAOT Publications ACE.

Christiansen, C., & Baum, C. (1997). Person-environment occupational performance: A conceptual model for practice. In C. H. Christiansen, & C. M. Baum, (Eds.), *Occupational therapy: Enabling function and well-being* (2nd ed., pp. 47-70). Thorofare NJ: Slack.

Clark, F. P. (1917). The beneficial effects of work therapy for the insane. *Modern Hospital, 8,* 392-393.

Connolly, K., & Dalgleish, M. (1989). The emergence of a tool-using skill in infancy. *Developmental Psychology*, *25*, 894-912.

Crepeau, E. B., & Schell, B. A. B. (2009). Analyzing occupational and activity. In E. B. Crepeau, E. S. Cohn, & B. A. B. Schell (Eds.), Willard & Spackman's occupational therapy (11th ed., pp. 359-373). Philadelphia: Lippincott Williams & Wilkins.

Doble, S. E., & Magill-Evans, J. (1992). A model of social interaction to guide occupational therapy practice. *Canadian Journal of Occupational Therapy, 59*, 141-150.

Dunn, W., Brown, C., & McGuigan, A. (1994). The ecology of human performance: A framework for considering the effect of the context. *American Journal of Occupational Therapy, 48,* 595-607.

Dunton, W. R. (1928). *Prescribing occupational therapy*. Springfield: Charles C. Thomas.

Einhorn, S. (2003). *Den sjunde dagen* [The seventh day]. Stockholm: MånPocket.

Englund, B. (1997). *BSI: Bedömning av social interaktion* (Version 2). [ASI: Assessment of Social Interaction]. Unpublished test manual, Umeå University, Sweden.

Englund, B., Bernspång, B., & Fisher, A. G. (1995). Development of an instrument for assessment of social interaction skills in occupational therapy. *Scandinavian Journal of Occupational Therapy*, *2*, 17-23.

Fearing, V. G., & Clark, J. (Eds.). (2000). Individuals in context: A practical guide to client-centered practice. Thorofare, NJ: Slack.

Fetters, L., & Kluzik, J. (1996). The effects of neurodevelopmental treatment versus practice on the reaching of children with spastic cerebral palsy. *Physical Therapy, 76,* 346-358.

Fisher, A.G. (1989). *Assessment of Motor and Process Skills* (Research ed.), unpublished test manual.

Fisher, A. G. (1994). Functional assessment and occupation: Critical issues for occupational therapy. *New Zealand Journal of Occupational Therapy*, *45*(2), 13-19.

Fisher, A. G. (1997). An expanded rehabilitative model of practice. In A. G. Fisher, *Assessment of Motor and Process Skills* (2nd ed., pp. 73-86). Fort Collins, CO: Three Star Press.

Fisher, A. G. (1998). Uniting practice and theory in an occupational framework, 1998 Eleanor Clarke Slagle Lecture. *American Journal of Occupational Therapy, 52,* 509-521.

Fisher, A. G. (2002/2006). *Occupational Therapy Intervention Process Model: A model for planning and implementing top–down, client-centered, and occupation-based occupational therapy*, unpublished manuscript.

Fisher, A. G. (2003). *Assessment of Motor and Process Skills. Vol. 1: Development, Standardization, and Administration Manual* (5th ed.). Fort Collins, CO: Three Star Press.

Fisher, A. G. (2006a). *Assessment of Motor and Process Skills. Vol. 1: Development, Standardization, and Administration Manual* (6th ed.). Fort Collins, CO: Three Star Press.

Fisher, A. G. (2006b). Overview of performance skills and client factors. In H. M. Pendleton, & W. Schultz-Krohn (Eds.), *Pedretti's occupational therapy: Practice skills for physical dysfunction* (6th ed., pp. 372-402). St. Louis MO: Mosby Elsevier.

Fisher, A. G. (2006c). *Assessment of Motor and Process Skills. Vol. 2: User Manual* (6th ed.). Fort Collins, CO: Three Star Press.

Fisher, A. G., Atler, K., & Potts, A. (2007). Effectiveness of occupational therapy with frail community living older adults. *Scandinavian Journal of Occupational Therapy, 14,* 240-249.

Fisher, A. G., Bryze, K., Hume, V, & Griswold, L. A. (2007). *School AMPS: School Version of the Assessment of Motor and Process Skills* (2nd ed.). Ft. Collins, CO: Three Star Press.

Fisher, A. G., & Griswold, L. A. (2009). *Evaluation of Social Interaction.* Ft. Collins, CO: Three Star Press.

Fisher, A. G., & Kielhofner, G. (1995). Skill in occupational performance. In G. Kielhofner, *A model of human occupation: Theory and application* (2nd ed., pp. 113-137). Baltimore: Williams & Wilkins.

Fisher, A. G., & Nyman, A. (2007). *OTIPM: En model för ett professionellt resonemang som främjar bästa praxis i arbetsterapi* (FOU-rapport 2007) [OTIPM: A model for professional reasoning that promotes best practice in occupational therapy]. Nacka, Sweden: Förbundet Sveriges Arbetsterapeuter.

Flinn, N. A., Jackson, J., Gray, J. M., & Zemke, R. (2008). Optimizing abilities and capacities: Range of motion, strength, and endurance. In M. V. Radomski & C. A. Trombly Latham (Eds.), *Occupational therapy for physical dysfunction* (6th ed.) (pp. 573-597). Philadelphia: Lippincott Williams & Wilkins.

Flinn, N. A., & Radomski, M. V. (2008). Learning. In M. V. Radomski & C. A. Trombly Latham (Eds.), *Occupational therapy for physical dysfunction* (6th ed.) (pp. 382-401). Philadelphia: Lippincott Williams & Wilkins.

Flinn, N. A., Trombly Latham, C. A., & Podolski, C. R.. (2008). Assessing abilities and capacities: Range of motion, strength, and endurance. In M. V. Radomski & C. A. Trombly Latham (Eds.), *Occupational therapy for physical dysfunction* (6th ed.) (pp. 91-185). Philadelphia: Lippincott Williams & Wilkins.

Fortmeier, S., & Thanning, G. (1998). Historien om Ole som råker ut för en olycka med sin surfbräda [The story of Ole who has an accident with his surfboard]. In S. Fortmeier & G. Thanning, *Sett med patientens ögon* [Seen with the patient's eyes] (pp. 20-28). Lund, Sweden: Studentlitteratur.

Förbundet Sveriges Arbetsterapeuter (2004). *FSAs kvalitetspolicy* [FSA's Quality Policy]. Retrieved October 20, 2008 from http://www.fsa.akademikerhuset.se

Förbundet Sveriges Arbetsterapeuter (2005). *Etisk kod: Berördas rättigheter* [Ethical code: Rights of the concerned]. Retrieved September 5, 2007 from http//www.fsa.akademikerhuset.se.

Greene, D. P., & Roberts, S. L. (2005). *Kinesiology: Movement in the context of activity* (2nd ed.). St. Louis: Mosby.

Gritzer, G., & Arluke, A. (1985). *The making of rehabilitation.* Berkeley: University of California Press.

Hagedorn, R. (1995). *Occupational therapy: Perspectives and processes.* Edinburgh, Scotland: Churchill Livingstone.

Hagedorn, R. (1997). *Foundations for practice in occupational therapy* (2nd ed.). New York: Churchill Livingstone.

Haugen, J. B., & Mathiowetz, V. (1995). Contemporary task-oriented approach. In C. A. Trombly (Ed.), *Occupational therapy for physical dysfunction* (4th ed., pp. 510-527). Baltimore: Williams & Wilkins.

Hutzler, Y., Chacham, A., Bergman, U., & Szeinberg, A. (1998). Effects of a movement and swimming program on vital capacity and water orientation skills of children with cerebral palsy. *Developmental Medicine and Child Neurology, 40,* 176-181.

Hällgren, M., & Kottorp, A., (2005). Effects of occupational therapy program in activities of daily living and awareness of disability in persons with intellectual disabilities. *Australian Occupational Therapy Journal, 52*, 350-359.

Individuals with Disabilities Education Improvement Act of 2004, Pub.L. No. 108–446, 20 U.S.C., 1400 et seq.

Jongbloed, L., Brighton, C., & Stacey, S. (1988). Factors associated with independent meal preparation, self-care and mobility in CVA clients. *Canadian Journal of Occupational Therapy*, *55*, 259-263.

Judge, J. O., Schechtman, K., Cress, E., & the FICSIT Group (1996). The relationship between physical performance measures and independence in instrumental activities of daily living. *Journal of the American Geriatrics Society*, *44*, 1332-1341.

Kaplan, B. J., Polatajko, H. J., Wilson, B. N., & Faris, P. D. (1993). Reexamination of sensory integration treatment: A combination of two efficacy studies. *Journal of Learning Disabilities, 26,* 342-347.

Kerr, T. (1999, February 8). Motivation in rehab: Getting — and keeping — your patients interested. *Advance for Occupational Therapists, 15,* 24-25.

Kielhofner, G. (1997). *Conceptual Foundations of Occupational Therapy* (2nd ed.). Philadelphia: F. A. Davis.

Kielhofner, G. (2002). A model of human occupation: Theory and application (3rd ed.). Philadelphia: Lippincott Williams & Wilkins.

Kielhofner, G. (2008). A model of human occupation: Theory and application (4th ed.). Philadelphia: Lippincott Williams & Wilkins.

Kielhofner, G., & Fisher, A. G. (1991). The mind-brain-body relationships. In A. G. Fisher, E. M. Murray, & A. C. Bundy (Eds.), *Sensory integration: Theory and practice* (pp. 27-45). Philadelphia: F. A. Davis.

Kottorp, A., Hällgren, M., Bernspång, B., & Fisher, A. G. (2003). Client-centred occupational therapy for persons with mental retardation: Implementation of an intervention programme in activities of daily living tasks. *Scandinavian Journal of Occupational Therapy, 10*, 51-60.

Law, M., Baptiste, S., Carswell, A., McColl, M. A., Polatajko, H., & Pollock, N. (2005). *Canadian Occupational Performance Measure* (4th ed.). Toronto, Ontario: Canadian Association of Occupational Therapists.

Law, M., Russell, D., Pollock, N., Rosenbaum, P., Walter, S., & King, G. (1997). A comparison of intensive neurodevelopmental therapy plus casting and a regular occupational therapy program for children with cerebral palsy. *Developmental Medicine and Child Neurology, 39,* 664-670.

Letts, S., Law, M., Rigby, P., Cooper, B., Stewart, S., & Strong, S. (1994). Person–environment assessments in occupational therapy. *American Journal of Occupational Therapy, 48,* 608-618.

Lichtenberg, P. A., & Nanna, M. (1994). The role of cognition in predicting activities of daily living and ambulation functioning in the oldest-old rehabilitation patients. *Rehabilitation Psychology, 39,* 251-262.

Lindstrom, P. R., & Westropp, J. (1999, March). Renewed energy following an epiphany at Annual Conference. *Gerontology Special Interest Quarterly, 22*(1), 1-3.

Llorens, L. A. (1993). Activity analysis: Agreement between participants and observers on perceived factors in occupation components. *Occupational Therapy Journal of Research, 13,* 198-211.

Ma, H., Trombly, C. A., & Robinson-Podolski, C. (1999). The effect of context on skill acquisition and transfer. *American Journal of Occupational Therapy, 53,* 138-144.

Mathiowetz, V., & Wade, M. G. (1995). Task constraints and functional motor performance of individuals with and without multiple sclerosis. *Ecological Psychology, 7,* 99-123.

Merriam-Webster (1996). *Merriam-Webster's collegiate dictionary* (10th ed.). Springfield MA: Author.

Mosey, A. C. (1981). *Occupational therapy: Configuration of a profession.* New York: Raven Press.

Mosey, A. C. (1986). *Psychosocial components of occupational therapy.* New York: Raven Press.

Munkholm, M. (2008, July). *Evaluating the effectiveness of a school-based occupational therapy program in Sweden.* Paper presented at the 2008 International Assessment of Motor and Process Skills (AMPS) Symposium: Measuring, Planning, and Implementing Occupation-based Programs. Halifax, Nova Scotia, Canada.

Nakayama, H., Jørgensen, H. S., Raaschou, H. O., & Olsen, T. S. (1994). Compensation in recovery of upper extremity function after stroke: The Copenhagen Stroke Study. *Archives of Physical Medicine and Rehabilitation, 75,* 852-857.

Neistadt, M. E. (1992). Occupational therapy treatments for constructional deficits. *American Journal of Occupational Therapy, 46,* 141-148.

Neistadt, M. E. (1995). Methods of assessing patients' priorities: A survey of adult physical dysfunction settings. *American Journal of Occupational Therapy, 49,* 428_436.

Occupational therapy in the general hospital. (1917). *Modern Hospital, 8,* 425-427.

Oxford English Dictionary (2nd. ed.). (1989). Oxford: Clarendon Press.

Pedretti, L. W., & Zoltan, B. (1990). *Occupational therapy: Practice skills for physical dysfunction* (3rd ed.). Philadelphia: Mosby.

Pincus, T., Callahan, L. F., Brooks, R. H., Fuchs, H. A., Olsen, N. J., & Kaye, J. J. (1989). Self-report questionnaire scores in rheumatoid arthritis compared with traditional physical, radiographic, and laboratory measures. *Annals of Internal Medicine*, *110*, 259-266.

Piper, W. (1930). *Little engine that could.* New York: Platt & Munk.

Price, P. (2009). The therapeutic relationship. In E. B. Crepeau, E. S. Cohn, & B. A. B. Schell (Eds.), Willard & Spackman's occupational therapy (11th ed., pp. 328-341). Philadelphia: Lippincott Williams & Wilkins.

Quiroga, V. A. M. (1995). *Occupational therapy: The first 30 years, 1900 to 1930.* Bethesda, MD: American Occupational Therapy Association.

Reed, B. R., Jagust, W. J., & Seab, J. P. (1989). Mental status as a predictor of daily function in progressive dementia. *Gerontologist*, *29*, 804-807.

Reed, K. L., & Sanderson, S. N. (1999). *Concepts of occupational therapy* (4th ed.). Philadelphia: Lippincott Williams & Wilkins.

Rogers, C. (1951). *Client-centered therapy: Its current practice, implications and theory*. London: Constable.

Shay, K. A., Duke, L. W., Conboy, T., Harrell, L. E., Callaway, R., & Folks, D. G. (1991). The clinical validity of the Mattis Dementia Rating Scale in staging Alzheimer's dementia. *Journal of Geriatric Psychiatry and Neurology*, *4*, 18-25.

Skurla, E., Rogers, J. C., & Sunderland, T. (1988). Direct assessment of activities of daily living in Alzheimer's disease: A controlled study. *Journal of the American Geriatrics Society*, *36*, 97-103.

Teri, L., Borson, S., Kiyak, H. A., & Yamagishi, M. (1989). Behavioral disturbance, cognitive dysfunction, and functional skill: Prevalence and relationship in Alzheimer's disease. *Journal of the American Geriatrics Society*, *37*, 109-116.

Three Star Press (2005). *Assessment of Motor and Process Skills computer-scoring program*. Fort Collins, CO: Author.

Tickle-Degnen, L. (2008). Therapeutic rapport. In M. V. Radomsky & C. A. Trombly (Eds.), *Occupational therapy for physical dysfunction* (6th ed.) (pp. 402-419). Philadelphia: Lippincott Williams & Wilkins.

Törnqvist, K., & Sonn, U. (2001). *ADL-Taxonomi: En bedömning av aktivitetsförmåga* [ADL Taxonomy: An evaluation of ADL ability]. Nacka, Sweden: Förbundet Sveriges Arbetsterapeuter

Trombly, C. (1993). The Issue Is — Anticipating the future: Assessment of occupational function. *American Journal of Occupational Therapy*, *47*, 253-257.

Trombly, C. A. (1995a). Occupation: Purposefulness and meaningfulness as therapeutic mechanisms, 1995 Eleanor Clarke Slagle Lecture. *American Journal of Occupational Therapy, 49,* 960-972.

Trombly, C. A. (1995b). Purposeful activity. In C. A. Trombly (Ed.), *Occupational therapy for physical dysfunction* (4th ed.) (pp. 237-253). Baltimore: Williams & Wilkins.

Trombly, C. A. (1995c). Retraining basic and instrumental activities of daily living. In C. A. Trombly (Ed.), *Occupational therapy for physical dysfunction* (4th ed.) (pp. 289-318). Baltimore: Williams & Wilkins.

Trombly, C. A. (1995d). Theoretical foundations for practice. In C. A. Trombly (Ed.), *Occupational therapy for physical dysfunction* (4th ed.) (pp. 15-27). Baltimore: Williams & Wilkins.

Trombly Latham, C. A. (2008a). Conceptual foundations of practice. In M. V. Radomski & C. A. Trombly Latham (Eds.), *Occupational therapy for physical dysfunction* (6th ed.) (pp. 1-20). Philadelphia: Lippincott Williams & Wilkins.

Trombly Latham, C. A. (2008b). Occupation as therapy: Selection, gradation, analysis, and adaption. In M. V. Radomski & C. A. Trombly Latham (Eds.), *Occupational therapy for physical dysfunction* (6th ed.) (pp. 358-401). Philadelphia: Lippincott Williams & Wilkins.

Trombly Latham, C. A. (2008c). Occupation: Philosophy and concepts. In M. V. Radomski & C. A. Trombly Latham (Eds.), *Occupational therapy for physical dysfunction* (6th ed.) (pp. 339-357). Philadelphia: Lippincott Williams & Wilkins.

Upham, E. G. (1917). Some principles of occupational therapy. *Modern Hospital, 8,* 409-413.

Watson, D. E. (1997). *Task analysis: An occupational performance approach.* Bethesda, MD: American Occupational Therapy Association.

Weiler, P. G., Chiriboga, D. A., & Black, S. A. (1994). Comparison of mental status tests: Implication for Alzheimer's patients and their caregivers. *Journal of Gerontology*, *49*, S44-51.

Whelihan, W. M., Emerson, L. L., Kleban, M. H., & Granick, S. (1984). Mental status and memory assessment as predictors of dementia. *Journal of Gerontology*, *39*, 572-576.

Wikipedia (2009). Develpmental dyspraxia. Retrieved March 6, 2009 from http://en.wikipedia.org/wiki/Developmental_dyspraxia.

World Health Organization (2001). *International classification of functioning, disability and health: ICF*. Geneva: Author.

Wu, C. Trombly, C. A., Lin, K., & Tickle-Degnan, L. (2000). A kinematic study of contextual effects on reaching performance in persons with and without stroke: Influences of object availability. *Archives of Physical Medicine and Rehabilitation, 81,* 95-101.

8. APPENDIX

8.1 Relationship between the Occupational Therapy Practice Framework and ICF

With the introduction of the first Occupational Therapy Practice Framework (Framework) (AOTA, 2002), there has been increasing discussion of the relationship between the Framework and ICF (WHO, 2001). Combined with this has been continued confusion related to the motor, process, and social interaction skills summarized in Chapter 6. That is, despite efforts to clearly present performance skills as the smallest observable units of occupational performance, ***not*** person factors and body functions, many occupational therapy authors continue to refer to them as if they were person factors and body functions. It is my hope, by including the equivalent ICF codes with the performance skills listed in Chapter 6, that this confusion will be eliminated. In an attempt to further clarify the difference between person factors and body functions, as defined in ICF, and performance skills, as defined in the OTIPM as well as in the original Framework and the Model of Human Occupation, their relationship is portrayed in Table 10. I have discussed elsewhere, in greater detail, the relationship among performance skills, the Framework, and ICF (Fisher, 2006b).

8.2 An Occupational Therapy Program Based on the OTIPM

In northern Sweden, occupational therapists working in the Västerbotten County Council (VLL) have recently been involved in the development of a general occupational therapy program based on the OTIPM. An occupational therapy program is a description of the evaluation, intervention, and reevaluation procedures for a group of patients (FSA, 2004). More specifically, an occupational therapy program provides the occupational therapist with a structure to ensure a systematic way of working. The program must also ***ensure that any structure developed is not so rigid as to preclude flexible, client-centered occupational therapy intervention programs that meet the needs of individual clients***.

Table 10 Relationship Between Occupational Therapy Practice Framework Domains of Practice (AOTA, 2002) (*italic*) and the World Health Organization's International Classification of Functioning, Disability, and Health (ICF) (WHO, 2001) (bold)

Activities and participation			Person factors and body functions and structures (*Client factors*)			Contextual factors
			Person factors and body functions			
Performance in areas of occupation	*Activities: task performances*	*Performance skills: smallest observable units of a task performance*	*Underlying ability*	*Performance component*	*Body structures*	*Context*
Self-care, Chapter 5 *Personal activities of daily living* (PADL) **Domestic life, Chapter 6** *Instrumental activities of daily living* (IADL) **Major life areas, Chapter 8** *Education, work* • Education • Work & employment • Economic life **Community, social, and civic life, Chapter 9** *Play, leisure* • Community life • Recreation & leisure • Religion & spirituality • Political life **Particular interpersonal relationships, Chapter 7** *Social participation* • Formal & informal • Family • Intimate	Putting on clothes Brushing one's teeth Eating a meal Preparing a glass of juice and a bowl of cereal Folding laundry Shopping Writing a story Coloring a picture Typing a memo Interviewing for a job Playing baseball Knitting a sweater Picking berries or mushrooms in the woods Interacting and relating to one's employer Socializing with friends at a party Caring for a child	**General tasks and demands, Chapter 2** *Process skills* • *Choosing* the correct shirt • *Gathering* crayons and paper to a table • *Organizing* papers on one's desk • *Initiating* swinging the baseball bat **Mobility, Chapter 4** *Motor skills* • *Lifting* a shirt • *Reaching* for a toothbrush • *Grasping* the baseball bat securely • *Running* to second base **Communication, Chapter 3 and General interpersonal interactions, Chapter 7** *Social interaction skills* • *Approaching* a partner and *starting* a conversation • *Turning toward* and *looking* at one's social partner • *Taking turns* with one's social partner • *Answering* questions with relevant replies **Learning and applying knowledge, Chapter 1** • Watching a baseball game • Listening to a lecture • Reading a book • Learning to manipulate a knife and fork	Remembering Developing a plan Sustaining attention Being aware of one's disability Regulating one's mood Enduring Lifting one's arm and reaching out Closing one's hand Executing coordinated movements Walking with a "normal" gait pattern Seeing Tasting Producing fluent speech Biting Chewing	**Mental, Chapter 1** • Memory • Cognition • Perception • Sustaining attention • Self-confidence • Insight • Motivation • Emotion **Cardiovascular and respiratory, Chapter 4** • Exercise tolerance • Aerobic capacity **Neuromusculoskeletal/ movement, Chapter 7** • Mobility of joints • Muscle power • Muscle tone (tension) • Control of voluntary movements • Gait pattern **Sensory/pain, Chapter 2** • Visual acuity • Sound discrimination **Voice and speech, Chapter 3** • Production of voice • Fluency of speech **Other body systems and the skin, Chapters 5, 6, 8**	**Brain and spinal cord** **Heart, lungs** **Bones, joints, muscles, and ligaments** **Eye and ear** **Nose, mouth, pharynx and larynx** **Stomach, glands, kidney, hair**	**Personal factors** *Personal* • Age and life stage (*temporal*) • Race/ethnicity • Gender • Sociocultural background • Educational background • Personality/character style • Habits and roles **Environmental factors** • **Products and technology** *Physical: objects, tools, devices* • **Natural environment and human made changes** *Physical: buildings and natural terrains* ▪ Spaces and settings ▪ Environmental features ▪ Day/night cycles (*temporal*) • **Support and relationships** *Social* ▪ Family ▪ Health care providers • **Attitudes, systems, and policies** *Cultural*

Occupational therapy programs are to be ***developed based on existing evidence and models of practice*** — ideally, models that are occupation-based. The former means that the specific evaluation, intervention, and reevaluation procedures are to be chosen based on evidence as to which ones are most effective with the particular group of clients in question. In the absence of published research, that evidence can come from systematic evaluation of program outcomes. That is, well designed occupational therapy programs also provide the ***foundation for developing systematic strategies for documentation, including measurable baselines, goals, and outcomes***. Systematic documentation enables the occupational therapist to generate measurable results that can be used for quality assurance and evidence-based practice. These, in turn, can provide the evidence needed to retain or discontinue procedures currently in the program.

The principal persons involved in the development of the general occupational therapy program were comprised of a working group and a reference group. The persons in the ***working group*** were: Christer Larsson (leader of program development within VLL), Agneta Carlsson, Marina Lycksell-Isaksson, Catrine Nygren, Pia Björk, and Anne G. Fisher. The ***reference group*** included the working group as well as the following persons: Jenny Larsson, Lena Eliasson, Anita Englund, Eva Enarsson, Lena Nygård, Birgitta Bernspång, and Gunilla Bergh. Together, they represented diverse clinical settings and client groups, as well as the academic occupational therapy education program. The general occupational therapy program was developed through a consensus process that also included input from additional occupational therapists within each group member's professional network.

The general occupational therapy program developed by this group of occupational therapists is ***intended to be used by others*** to create specific programs for individual settings and client groups. Therefore, ***the general program included on the following pages may be copied, altered, or used in any way that will help occupational therapists ensure quality occupational therapy services***. What is critical is that the specific occupational programs developed based on this one specify (a) what services the occupational therapist will offer, and (b) how the occupational therapist will implement each phase. Phases that are not included as part of the occupational therapy services provided within a given setting are to be eliminated.

The program is described in Table 11. This table includes two levels of "What" columns that reflect the phases of the intervention process. The "How" column provides more concrete descriptions of how we are to practice. Also included are the following:

1. ***Questions to answer*** — questions that the occupational therapist can ask him- or herself. They are intended to guide the occupational therapist's reasoning. They are *not* questions to be posed to the client.

2. ***It has to do with*** — further clarification, added when needed to clarify what it is that we are to do at that phase.

3. ***Some examples of instruments*** — representative examples of standardized and nonstandardized methods the occupational therapist may choose to use.

The occupational therapy process that accompanies the program description (see Figures 17 to 19) clarifies further what is to be documented at each phase in the process. More specifically, the ***larger rectangle-shaped text boxes*** (e.g., *Inform about occupational therapy*) represent what the occupational therapist is to do. The specific details of what the occupational therapist is to do are to be documented in the occupational therapy program description (e.g., Table 11, although this program is still generic and needs to be modified to fit specific practice settings and client groups). The ***smaller dark squares*** specify that there is something to be documented, and the ***text below the small dark squares*** indicates what is to be documented.

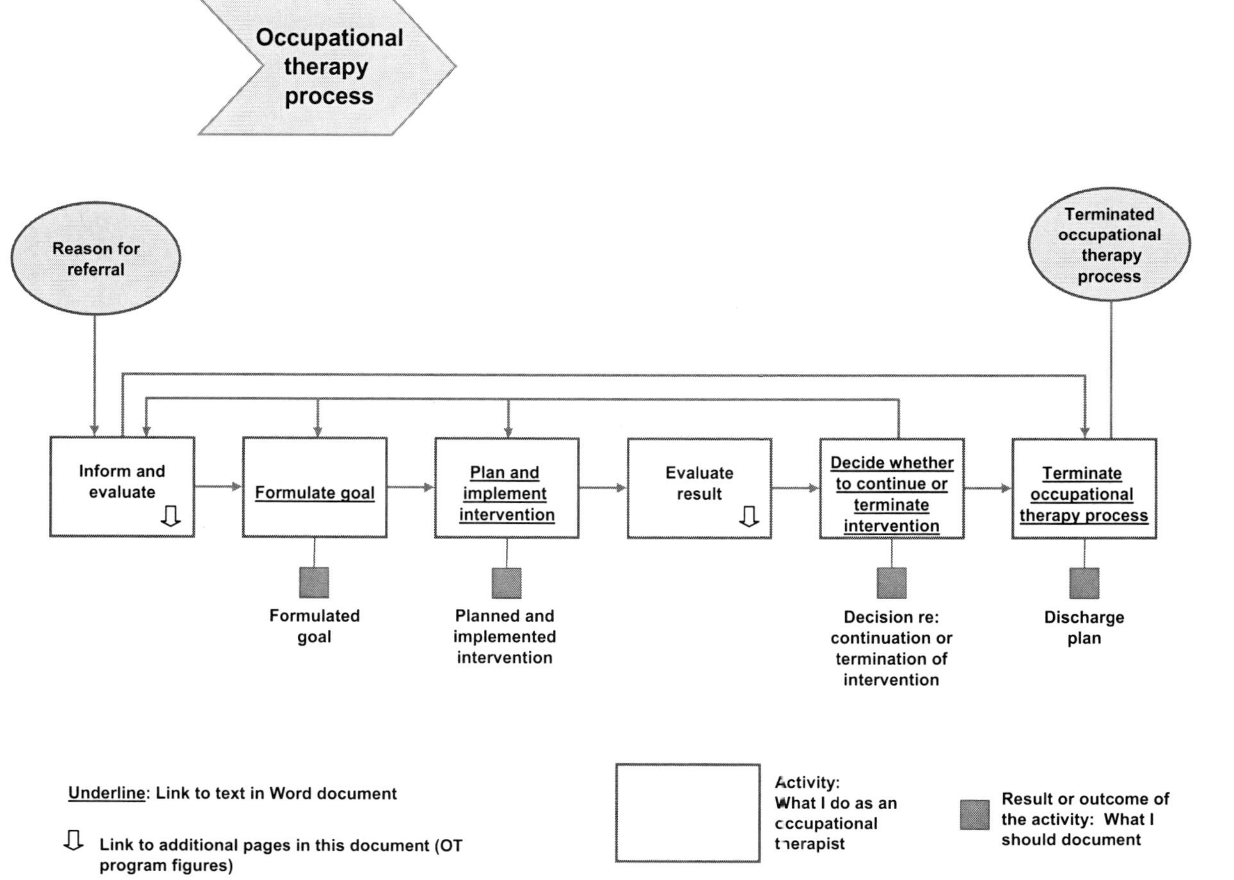

Figure 17. **Schematic representation of the occupational therapy process, showing activities (what the occupational therapists is to do) and results (what is to be documented). The small white arrows indicate links to Figures 18 and 19, which show those phases in more detail.**

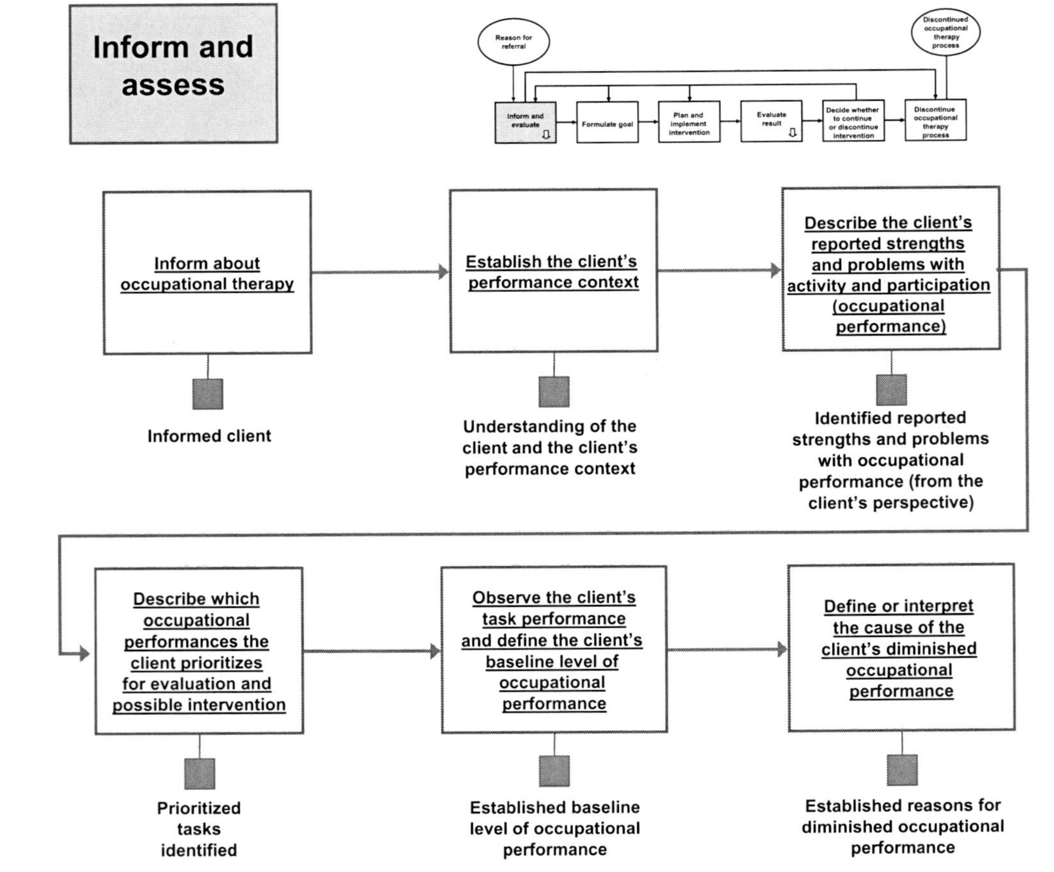

Figure 18. **Schematic representation of the *Inform and assess* (evaluation) phase of the occupational therapy process. Figure 17 is shown at the top of the figure so as to clarify where this phase fits in the overall process.**

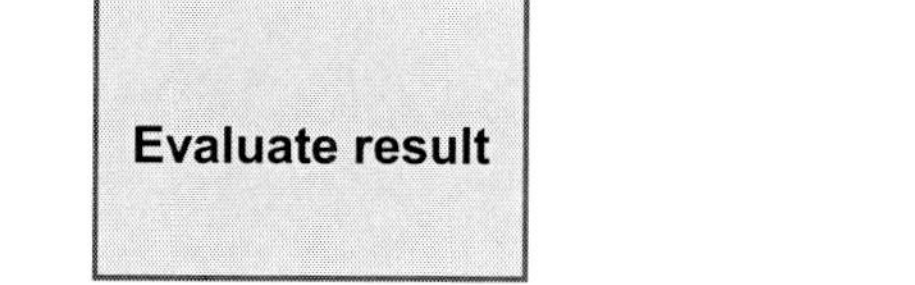

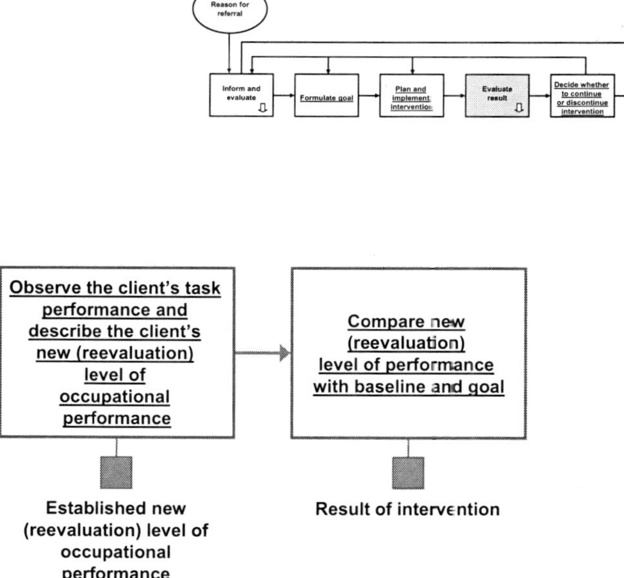

Underline: Link to text i Word document

General occupational therapy program for Västerbotten County Council, 23 January, 2008

Figure 19. **Schematic representation of the *Evaluate result* (reevaluation) phase of the occupational therapy process. Figure 17 is shown at the top of the figure so as to clarify where this phase fits in the overall process.**

Table 11 A General Occupational Therapy Program Based on the OTIPM

What	*What*	*How*
Inform and assess	Inform about occupational therapy	➢ Oral and/or written presentation to the client (e.g., person, client constellation), using the occupational therapist's own words • Questions to answer: o Is the client informed about: ▪ What is occupational therapy? ▪ What we have as our focus at this workplace/department? ▪ What is our unique role? ▪ What we can offer?
Inform and assess	Establish the client's performance context	➢ Interview with the client (i.e., person and/or others in the client constellation) and other professionals and Review of existing documentation • Questions to answer: o Who is the client? o What are the client's needs? o What tasks does the client want and/or need to perform? o In what environments? • It has to do with: o Identifying aspects of the following dimensions that support and limit performance of daily life tasks: ▪ Person factors (e.g., goals, values, habits, interests, roles, first impression of physical and psychological body functions), ▪ The physical environment, ▪ The social environment (e.g., people, quality of relationships, collaboration with others) ▪ Institutional/cultural factors (e.g., economy, shared values, rules/regulations, norms) • Some examples of instruments: o Documented "home grown" interview guide o School Function Assessment (SFA)

What	***What***	***How***
Inform and assess	Describe the client's reported strengths and problems with activity and participation (occupational performance)	➢ Interview with the client (i.e., person and/or others in the client constellation) • Questions to answer: o What tasks does the client experience as strengths and/or support engagement in life roles? o What tasks does the client experience problems and/or limit engagement in life roles? • Some examples of instruments: o Documented "home grown" interview guide o ADL-Taxonomy o Canadian Occupational Performance Measure (COPM) o Occupational Self Assessment OSA) ***Note***. Documentation of supports and limitations related to person factors and/or the environment are discussed above.
Inform and assess	Describe which occupational performances the client prioritizes for evaluation and possible intervention	➢ Interview with the client (i.e., person and/or others in the client constellation) • Question to answer: o What task performances does the client prioritize? • Some examples of instruments: o Documented "home grown" interview guide o ADL-Taxonomy o Canadian Occupational Performance Measure (COPM) o Occupational Self Assessment (OSA)

What	*What*	*How*
Inform and assess	Observe the client's task performance and define the client's baseline level of occupational performance	➢ Observation of performance of those tasks the client (e.g., person and/or others in the client constellation) has prioritized, Or, if observation is not possible, interview regarding quality of performance • Question to answer: o What is the quality of the client's performance of prioritized tasks? • It has to do with: o Evaluation of the client's global quality of task performance and/or the quality of the smallest observable units of occupational performance (e.g., motor, process, social interaction skills). o Based on the occupational therapist's evaluation, define and describe the actions of performance that were observed to be effective or ineffective (e.g., time/space inefficient, physically effortful, requiring assistance, unsafe, socially inappropriate); and/or, based on the client's verbalization, were reported to be unsatisfactory, painful, etc. • Some examples of instruments: o Documented "home grown" observation guide o Assessment of Motor and Process Skills (AMPS) o School Version of the Assessment of Motor and Process Skills (School AMPS) o Evaluation of Social Interaction (ESI) o Assessment of Communication and Interaction Skill (ACIS) ➢ Define baseline level of occupational performance • A baseline is a measurable/observable description of: o What task the client performed, and o With what quality and/or support/assistance the client performed the task ***Note***. Do not use the words *problem* or *difficulty* in the definition of a baseline. Example baseline statements: *"When observed preparing a cooked meal (chicken, boiled potatoes, broccoli, sauce, and a beverage), he needed several verbal cues. He took more than 10 short pauses, he used four different workspaces, and he demonstrated mild physical clumsiness."* *"She needed physical assistance from two persons to get into the bathroom, and to transfer from her wheelchair to the toilet. She needed physical assistance from one person to remove and put on her clothing, and to wipe herself. Both she and her husband were dissatisfied with her need for help from others."*

What	*What*	*How*
Inform and assess	Define or interpret the cause of the client's diminished occupational performance	➢ Analysis of client's underlying body functions, personal factors, or environmental factors that limit the client's occupational performance • Questions to answer: o What are the possible causes? ▪ Person factors (e.g., goals, values, habits, interests, roles, first impression of physical and psychological body functions), ▪ The physical environment, ▪ The social environment (e.g., people, quality of relationships/collaboration with others) ▪ Institutional/cultural factors (e.g., economy, shared values, rules/regulations, norms) • It has to do with: o Taking into consideration the information that was gathered when the client's performance context was established o Reflecting back on the observation of the client's task performance and implement an activity analysis to identify cause o Implement additional evaluations using interview or instruments o Obtain information from evaluations performed by other professionals • Some examples of instruments: o ADL-focused Occupation-based Neurobehavioral Evaluation (A-ONE) o Assessment of Awareness of Disability (AAD) o Occupational Performance History Interview (OPHI-II) o Housing Enabler o Goniometer o Grip-It o Test of Visual Perceptual Skills (TVPS) o Mini-Mental State Exam (MMSE)

<table>
<tr><th>What</th><th>What</th><th>How</th></tr>
<tr><td>Formulate goal</td><td></td><td>➢ In collaboration with client (i.e., person and/or others in the client constellation), formulate the client's goal

• A goal is a measureable/observable description of:
  o What task the client wants do be able to perform
  o With what quality and/or support/assistance the client will be able to perform the task
  o When the client will be able to perform the task
Note. Do not use the words problem or difficulty in the definition of a goal.

• It has to do with:
  o Formulating the goal based on the tasks the client prioritized
  o Creating a description based on the client's desired quality of occupational performance:
    ▪ Time/space efficiency,
    ▪ Physical effort,
    ▪ Need for assistance,
    ▪ Safety,
    ▪ Social appropriateness,
    ▪ Satisfaction and/or
    ▪ Pain

Examples of goals:
"He will independently, without small pauses, and using only one workspace, prepare a cooked meal (e.g., baked salmon, boiled potatoes, salad, and beverage); he will continue to demonstrate mild physical clumsiness."

"She will, with assistance from her husband, manage toileting at a level with which both she and her husband express satisfaction."</td></tr>
</table>

What	*What*	*How*
Plan and implement intervention		➢ Collaborate with the client (i.e., person and/or others in the client constellation) to identify different alternatives for intervention and existing evidence • Questions to answer: o What possibilities for intervention exist? o For which interventions is there evidence? o What interventions does the client suggest? ➢ Choose a model for intervention: • Compensatory model, with the following interventions: o Using assistive devices and technology o Learning alternative methods for doing o Modifying the physical environment o Modifying the social environment o Educating and providing consultation to the person and/or others in the client constellation related to the above • Model for occupational skills training o Regain previous or develop new occupational skills so as to perform tasks in the same way as previously (or as do others), without use of compensatory strategies. Intervention is focused directly on occupational performance, with or without the use of grading or modifying the task challenge or complexity o Educate and provide consultation to the person and/or others in the client constellation related to the above • Model for training of person factors or body functions o Restore previous or develop new person factors or body functions o Educate and provide consultation to the person and/or others in the client constellation related to the above ***Note***. Even when this model is chosen, the client's goal remains occupation-focused, and interventions are implemented primarily occupation-based • Educational model o Inform and educate groups about occupation through: ▪ Seminars/lectures/workshops for client groups ▪ Seminars/lectures/workshops for family and significant others ▪ Seminars/lectures/workshops for care personnel

What	*What*	*How*
Plan and implement intervention (continued)		• Questions to answer: o What is the intervention plan? o What interventions were implemented?
Evaluate result	Observe the client's task performance and describe the client's new (reevaluation) level of occupational performance	➢ Observation of performance of those tasks the client (i.e., person and/or others in the client constellation) has prioritized, Or, if observation is not possible, interview regarding quality of performance • Question to answer: o What is the quality of the client's performance of prioritized tasks? • It has to do with: o Evaluation of the client's global quality of task performance and/or the quality of the smallest observable units of occupational performance (e.g., motor, process, social interaction skills) o Based on the occupational therapist's evaluation, define and describe the actions of performance that were observed to be effective or ineffective (e.g., time/space inefficient, physically effortful, requiring assistance, unsafe, socially inappropriate); and/or, based on the client's verbalization, were reported to be unsatisfactory, painful, etc. • Some examples of instruments: o Documented "home grown" observation guide o Assessment of Motor and Process Skills (AMPS) o School Version of the Assessment of Motor and Process Skills (School AMPS) o Evaluation of Social Interaction (ESI) o Assessment of Communication and Interaction Skill (ACIS) ➢ Define new (reevaluation) level of occupational performance • The new (reevaluation) level of performance is a measurable/observable description of: o What task the client performed, and o With what quality and/or support/assistance the client performed the task ***Note***. Do not use the words *problem* or *difficulty* in the definition of a new (reevaluation) level of performance

What	*What*	*How*
(continued)	(continued)	Examples of new (reevaluation) levels of performance: *"He reports that he can prepare a cooked meal (e.g., chicken, boiled potatoes, broccoli, sauce, and a beverage. He still needs occasional verbal assistance. He takes only two to three small pauses, and organizes tools and materials within only one workspace. As expected, he continues to demonstrate mild physical clumsiness.* *"She is able, with physical assistance from her husband, transfer from her wheelchair or bed to a commode, and get into the bathroom. She continues to require assistance from her husband to manage her clothing and wipe herself. Her husband expresses dissatisfaction as he now experiences back pain."*

Evaluate result	Compare new (reevaluation) level of performance with baseline and goal	➢ In collaboration with client (i.e., person and/or others in the client constellation), evaluate the result
		
		• Questions to answer:
		  o What differences exist between the baseline and new (reevaluation) level of performance?
		  o What differences exist between the goal and new (reevaluation) level of performance?
		  o To what extent was the goal reached?
		  o If the goal was not met, why not?
		
		Examples of results:
		"He partially met his goal."
		or
		"He did not meet his goal."
		
		"She partially met her goal; her husband misjudged his physical capacity."
		or
		"She did not meet her goal; her husband misjudged his physical capacity."

Decide whether to continue or terminate intervention		➢ In collaboration with client (i.e., person and/or others in the client constellation), determine whether intervention will be continued or terminated
		
		• Question to answer:
		  o Which alternative is chosen?:
		    ▪ Return to a step within "Inform and Assess"
		    ▪ Formulate a new goal
		    ▪ Retain the current goal(s) and select new interventions or continue with current interventions
		    ▪ Terminate the occupational therapy process

What	*What*	*How*
Terminate the occupational therapy process		➢ In collaboration with client (i.e., person and/or others in the client constellation), determine whether referral will be made for further occupational therapy • Questions to answer: o Where will further occupational therapy be implemented? o What is the purpose of further occupational therapy? o If there is a need for collaboration with others, with whom?